Gardening *for a* Lifetime

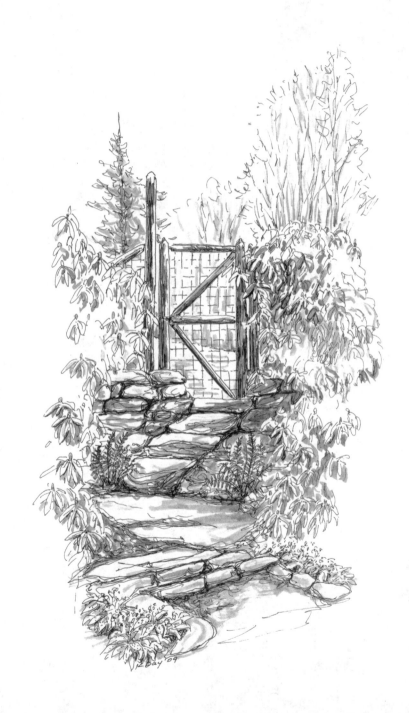

Gardening *for a* Lifetime

How to Garden Wiser As You Grow Older

By Sydney Eddison

Illustrations by
Kimberly Day Proctor

Timber Press
Portland ⚥ London

New paperback edition published in 2011 by Timber Press, Inc.

The Haseltine Building
133 S.W. Second Avenue, Suite 450
Portland, Oregon 97204-3527
www.timberpress.com

2 The Quadrant
135 Salusbury Road
London NW6 6RJ
www.timberpress.co.uk

ISBN: 978-1-60469-266-2 (pbk)
Printed in the United States of America

The Library of Congress has cataloged the hardcover edition as follows:

Eddison, Sydney, 1932–
    Gardening for a lifetime : how to garden wiser as you grow older /
by Sydney Eddison.
        p. cm.
    Includes index.
    ISBN 978-1-60469-065-1
    1. Gardening for older people. 2. Low maintenance gardening. I. Title.
    SB457.4.A34E33 2010
    635—dc22
                                                                        2009046594

A catalog record for this book is also available from the British Library.

In memory of my husband,
John Martin Ryalls Eddison

Contents

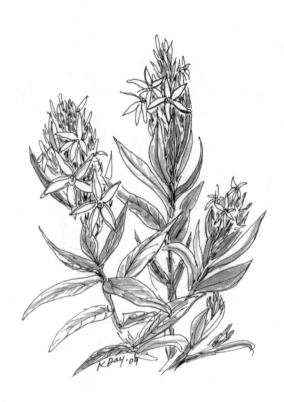

Acknowledgments

WRITERS ARE ADVISED to write about what they know. I've taken that advice to heart and written, yet again, about my own garden. As the garden is central to my life and happiness and to the book, its ongoing maintenance is critical. But without Erica Carroll, it might not have been possible. I have been physically unable to garden for the last five months.

Nevertheless, this remarkable young woman, who comes for only six hours a week, has managed the entire garden all season, with less-than-regular help from a college student. She found her own pace, set priorities, and never let one area take up time at the expense of another. For what she has done, I admire and cherish her and am deeply in her debt.

Almost as vital to the garden and the book has been the help of Terence Farrell and his young family. In the grip of the gardening passion, Terence is busy making his own garden, which will one day be admired and visited by many. But he has also volunteered in mine for the last two seasons, more than once bringing a friend from work, Georgia Shafer-Suriani. Terence has also been pressed into service for his computer skills, and his long-suffering wife, Rosa, and seven-year-old twins have put up with it all. My gratitude to the Farrells is boundless.

A Master Gardener with his own gardening business, Larry Birch volunteered to deliver three yards of topsoil and twelve yards of mulch, and to shovel it off his truck. He also transported topsoil to the woodland garden, where he weeded and planted primroses. What kindness!

To help me deadhead the daylilies this season, friends have

shown up every night, unbidden: Marilyn Rennagel, Lorie Barber, and Jane Hellman. For this kind service, my undying affection and so many thanks.

Having Anne Harrigan appear, more or less out of the blue, was an incredible stroke of luck. Anne, too, came as a volunteer and stayed on as my assistant and problem solver. I couldn't cope without her. For a few hours a week, she is a helpful bright spot in my life.

Martin and I had been devoted to Kim Proctor and her husband, David, for twenty years. We enjoyed watching their children grow up; Kim brought her mother to see my garden; and I know Kim's sister and a brother. So I feel that I know her whole family. I have always admired Kim's horticultural knowledge and loved her drawings, which appeared in the Oliver Nurseries catalog for years. She was the perfect partner on a book that is so close to my heart. Her sensitivity and compassion have made her a joy to work with, and her drawings say eloquently what I may have failed to express adequately in words.

I am also exceedingly fortunate to have Jane Dystel as my agent. She cares about her clients, treats their work with respect, and goes to great pains to see that it is presented in the best possible form. I appreciate the work that she and the staff of Dystel & Goderich Literary Management put into a proposal. Thanks for everything.

To Tom Fischer and Timber Press, more thanks for taking on this book. I'm lucky to have you.

And last but certainly not least, Gregory Piotrowski prepared the plant index and spared me embarrassment by a preliminary reading of the manuscript with an eye to the accuracy of botanical nomenclature. A 1986 graduate of the New York Botanical Garden School of Professional Horticulture, Greg stayed on as a gardener, and we met shortly thereafter. I have presumed upon this old and valued friendship before, so thanks yet again, Greg.

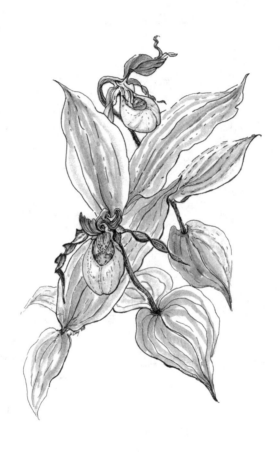

Preface

GARDENS AND GARDENERS age and change. Why wouldn't they? The passage of time brings about changes in all living things, yet old age always takes us by surprise. I'm stunned by it. In the sliding glass doors to the kitchen, I catch glimpses of an old woman hobbling around my garden, and I realize in amazement that it's me. When I began writing this book, I wasn't hobbling. That has happened during the last few months.

"The old order changeth, yielding place to new, / And God fulfils himself in many ways, lest one good custom should corrupt the world." When I was young and read Alfred Lord Tennyson's *Idylls of the King*, I rebelled against the idea that any good thing could possibly corrupt the world. How could it? And how could Arthur, that model of goodness, corrupt anything? But in a garden, it becomes quite clear. Change is nature's way of managing it all—animal, vegetable, and even mineral. The sands of the desert shift and mountains erode. Everything changes, and somehow or other it all works.

It's hard to say whether a garden is a metaphor for life or the other way around. Certainly, each phase of my life has been clearly reflected not only in the glass doors but also through them. The view today is very different from the same view in 1961. At that time, the kitchen was just a covered porch surrounded by long grass and brush. The glass doors were not put in until 1980, when there was finally something to see.

The garden emerged by fits and starts over a period of many years. But it doesn't seem so long ago that it was in its infancy and I was young. Now we are both old. The first rhododendrons I planted have trunks like trees, and a Chinese chestnut given to me as a sprout in a four-inch pot has reached a height of thirty-five feet.

Evidence of change is everywhere, in both garden and gardener. We've been through a lot together: the year the trees were defoliated by inch worms that hung in masses from their bare branches; drought years, when my husband and I pumped gray water from the bathtub to revive the wilting shrubs; a three-year plague of voles that decimated the shade plantings.

To balance these relatively minor setbacks, there have been so many moments of heart-stopping wonder and delight, such as the triumph of a yellow lady's slipper's first bloom. I now have a whole clump, and they remind me of my youth and the farmer

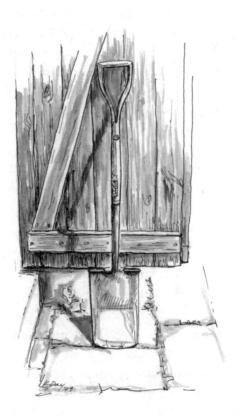

who taught me about wildflowers. He used to send away for plants and seed and managed to establish a small colony of yellow lady's slippers in the woods behind his farm.

My garden is full of wonderful memories. In April, I look forward every year to the poignant beauty of primroses planted in memory of my English mother. And in the summer, I think of Helen and Johnny Gill, my gardening mentors, who are responsible for the river of lamb's ears in front of the long perennial border.

For forty-eight years, the garden has been part of my life every day, in every season and in all weathers. It has witnessed my greatest joys and absorbed my deepest sorrows. It is a place of safety and comfort, an old forgiving friend who is always there for me, who protects and embraces me.

I cannot leave this place. It is where my husband and I spent a lifetime together and where I want to stay. The determination to remain here fueled my desire to find a simpler way to garden and to write about it. In addition, there were the letters I received after an article for *Fine Gardening* on reducing maintenance in the garden came out. Those letters have kept me in front of the computer.

This is my story and it is for my husband, but it is also for the kind people who wrote those letters. They told me a little bit about their stories, and as it turns out, we are all doing exactly the same thing—trying to hang on to something we love. And sometimes we feel that we are winning. Already, some of the strategies I've tried are working, and caring for the garden has become easier. So many gardeners will eventually find themselves in the same boat that I think our experiences worth sharing.

But first, a backward glance at the way the garden used to be. Because unless you know something of its history, you will not understand the significance of all the changes, voluntary and involuntary, that have taken place in recent years.

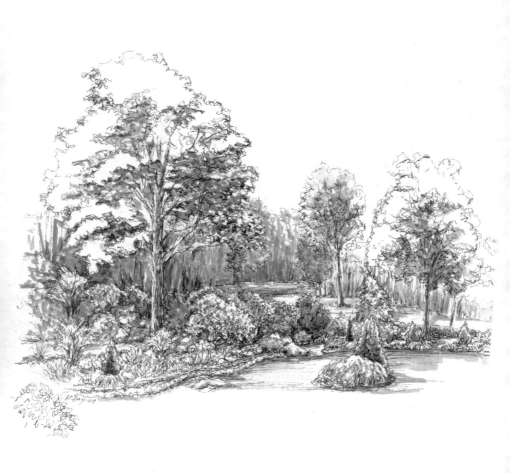

1

A Look Backward:
Tracing the Garden's History

It took a great deal of time and energy to make the garden as hard to manage as it ultimately became, and I loved every minute of it: every hour spent digging beds and planting shrubs, trees, and perennials; and all the countless more hours of pruning, dividing, and moving the plants around. It has been wonderful, and given the opportunity I would do the same all over again.

Gardeners garden the way they do because of the people they are, so in this chapter you will get to know me and my nongardening husband. He maintained that the reason we got on so well was that we had absolutely nothing in common. Certainly, we were the odd couple, but we were also a good team.

Martin was a lovely man with more patience than Job, a wicked wit, and a gentle nature. He grew up in Yorkshire, England, where his mother had a beautiful garden. While he admired it and always waxed nostalgic about the sweet peas that grew against its brick walls, he hadn't the least desire to work in the garden. Manual labor simply wasn't his idea of fun, and he was baffled by my enthusiasm for what seemed to him drudgery.

As an engineer, he designed machines to spare the human body. It was, therefore, inconceivable to him that any sane person could delight in digging holes, prying up boulders, and shoving rocks around. But I liked the exercise and the way my body felt at the end of the day. It was bliss to soak in a hot bath and think about the next unwieldy project—maybe clearing the field on the other side of the stone wall or adding a few more feet to the ever-lengthening perennial borders.

Thus, over the years, the garden took shape, and predictably my long-suffering spouse helped me. Although Martin never dug, planted, or pruned, he was a genius with gasoline engines and could get the best out of any piece of power equipment. Even an ancient Gravely tractor was persuaded to purr like a kitten and with it we cleared about two acres. He cut down the invasive barberry and bush honeysuckle with the tractor; I grubbed out the roots with the mattock, a tool like a blunt pickax with a stout handle.

Little by little, we unveiled old fieldstone walls that had been completely hidden by brush and poison ivy. Dilapidated but still beautiful, they became the boundaries of the garden. The flowing landscape within did not lend itself to arbitrary subdivision. So instead of "garden rooms," the nature of the plantings and the use of each area were determined by its topography. There was no plan. The garden developed according to the limitations of the site, our time, and a feel for the natural landscape.

The highest point lies to the west, where the remains of an old mountain chain runs north to the Berkshire Hills and south to the Appalachian Mountains. From our rocky, wooded ridge, the land drops steeply at first, then more gently, until it levels out behind the house. This relatively flat stretch became the upper lawn.

On the east, the lawn is bounded by a juniper hedge, which disguises an abrupt change in grade. Below the hedge, another plateau extends from the house toward the old red barn, which our predecessors used as a garage. The rest of the area they made into lawn and planted a number of fruit trees.

When we bought the property, only two aging apples and two young ones—a Macintosh and a Baldwin—remained. The old trees soon died, but the young ones prospered. Both must be fifty years old by now and have become handsome specimens. Beneath the spreading limbs of the Macintosh, we put down a circle of hardwood mulch and set up a picnic table. In the summer, it's a perfect place to have lunch.

On this lower level, the garden is cool, green, and undemanding. There are no flower beds, just the apple trees. Along the access road into the state forest, a thick, informal hedge of forsythia shuts out the world. Not that the world has ever intruded much on our privacy. Only a few cars go into the eight-hundred-acre tract of woodland that surrounds us.

Most of my serious gardening takes place around the perimeter of the upper lawn, where a long, curving perennial border follows the contours of the site. It was a happy accident that the slope improved drainage and that the eastern exposure suited a wide variety of hardy perennials. Begun in 1963 and extended by a few feet every year, the border crept along at the foot of the

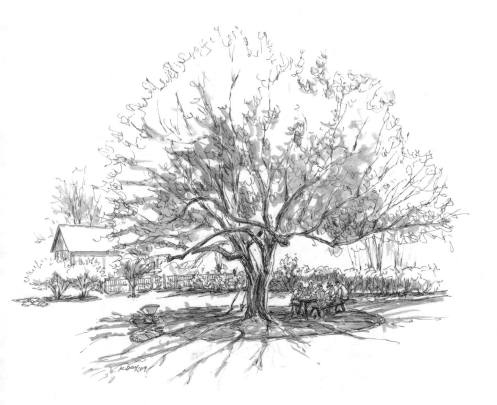

slope until it measured a hundred feet in length and fifteen to twenty feet in width.

At about the same pace, we tamed the hillside behind the border, getting rid of grapevines, poison ivy, barberries, and honeysuckle and excavating a dump full of old bed springs and rusted farm equipment. As we went along, I planted the rhododendrons that now provide an evergreen backdrop for the perennials.

The far end of the upper lawn is partially enclosed by two newer beds. Through the opening between them, you can see a bit of lovely old stone wall, and beyond the wall, what was once an open, sunny field. We cleared it in 1965, and for many years thereafter Martin mowed it three or four times during the growing season. In those days it looked like a park. But the hilly terrain made mowing with the Gravely hard work, and in time he mowed less often.

Inevitably, seeds from the surrounding trees took hold at the edges of the clearing, and saplings grew up on either side. Protected by the walls from the blades of the mower, these eventually became substantial trees. Today, they stretch their upper limbs across the clearing, reaching toward the light and each other. Shade is reclaiming the field.

Behind the long border, shade is also engulfing the hillside of rhododendrons. But they still get enough morning sun to flower abundantly. Once the size of bushel baskets, they are now huge mounds of gleaming foliage smothered in the spring with clouds of pink, red, and white blossoms.

Every year for thirty years, I expanded my domain and my horizons. By the 1970s I had begun to meet other gardeners, join plant societies, and take courses at the New York Botanical Garden. Inspired by these new influences, I became more ambitious, and the garden more complex, more interesting, and a great deal more work. Although Martin was unfailingly supportive, he had seen the writing on the wall. In a few years, I was madly casting around for help.

A series of teenage boys proved more entertaining than helpful, but at last I found Louise Marston. A contemporary and a
superb gardener, Lou came to me for three hours a week and introduced me to the miracle of mulch. Every year since, the flower
beds have received a blanket of leaves, harvested in the fall and
spread over the soil in the spring. You will be hearing more about
the time-saving benefits of mulch in another chapter.

Lou was followed by tousle-headed Ann Prentiss, young,
hardworking, and strong of limb. In 1990, the two of us removed the sod, dug out the rocks, and amended the soil for the
new flower beds at the far end of the upper lawn. But the sunny
climes of California beckoned, and Ann moved on, fortunately
not before introducing me to her friend Diane Campbell.

For the next nine years, Diane came for half a day a week.
Despite her slender build—everything about her was long, lean,
and elegant—she was a powerhouse in the garden. She and I
made the new borders wider and refined the lines of all the beds.
In the woodland garden, we extended the path until it com-

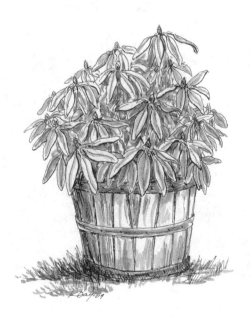

pletely encircled the pond and planted more and more primroses. Diane loved the woodland garden.

Meanwhile, I had written a book about making the garden,
and readers began to ask if they could come and see it. Dazzled
by the prospect of showing off our handiwork, Diane and I re-
doubled our efforts. Visitors did come and for a few shining seasons, the garden looked as close to perfect as a garden ever gets—
perennial borders neatly mulched, weedless, and crisply edged.

Then one spring, Diane began to look tired. We were con-
cerned, but she insisted that she was fine and went right on working. However, she did admit to occasionally feeling dizzy and
persuaded her younger sister, Deata Bertrand, to drive her over
from New York state where they both lived. At first, Deata served

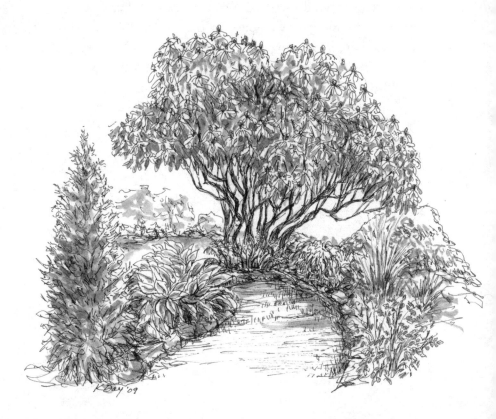

as Diane's go-fer, but she proved to be as capable and talented as her sister.

The Bertrand sisters were an extraordinary pair. Although neither had any training in horticulture, they were gifted gardeners, incredibly hard workers, and very good company. Martin and I were devoted to them, and Diane's sudden death, much too young, in 1999 came as a dreadful shock.

For another four years, Deata carried on, often bringing with her Ross Tanner, her next-door neighbor with whom she shared a vegetable garden. Ross helped with everything, quietly taking over the mowing from Martin, who no longer had the energy. But the day finally came when Ross, a retired telephone repairman, began to feel his age, too, and Deata simply could not afford the commitment of time. It was an hour's drive each way and hard work in between.

The truth was finally beginning to sink in. With the help of first Lou, then Ann, the remarkable Bertrand sisters, and Ross, I had created a garden that was impossible to maintain without assistance. These kind people had allowed me the illusion that I was still taking care of my garden. But I had been living in a fool's paradise. Without them, I couldn't possibly have managed. By this time, I was no spring chicken and in the future would need even more help, probably more than Martin and I could afford.

❧ GLEANINGS ❧

❧ Gardener, know thyself

My garden became as hard to manage as it did because I was a perfectionist, infatuated with a style and scale of perennial gardening suitable only for the relatively young and very energetic. For the first twenty-five years I got away with it, but ultimately I needed help to maintain my creation.

❧ Recognizing the problem

To need help should have been a warning sign in itself, but I ignored it. Instead, with the assistance of the wonderful people I found, I gleefully expanded the garden. In those days, three or fours hours of help a week was adequate and affordable.

❧ The wake-up call

What finally got my attention was the discovery that I had made a garden I couldn't possibly keep up without more help than my spouse and I could afford. On the other hand, I knew that sweeping changes would be even more expensive and could very likely make matters worse. So I didn't know what to do.

❧ The decision to change

Making the decision to change habits of a lifetime is hard enough, but to actually do it is harder. However, songwriter Johnny Mercer had the answer: "Something's gotta give." And I knew it.

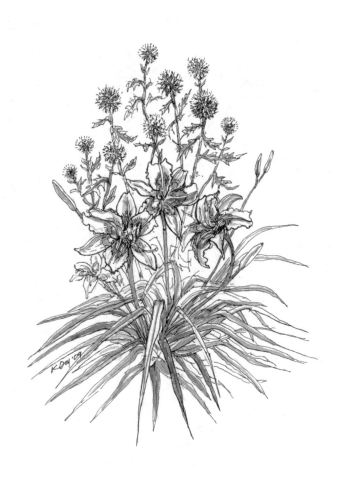

2

Changes:
Rethinking the Perennial Borders

WITH THE APPROACH of spring 2004, anxiety about the garden's future blossomed into panic. By May, the lawn was already a foot high, weeds were popping up everywhere, and the perennial borders were crying out for attention. I needed help soon or the garden would get completely out of hand. I also needed to bring my garden dreams into line with the realities of my life— diminished energy, less time, and a limited budget. Pondering ways to accomplish this feat, I considered reducing the area under cultivation but quickly abandoned that approach.

Settled into the embrace of the old stone walls, the garden is the size it needs to be in order to fill its setting. Nor did I see much point in sacrificing any of the beds. They all serve a purpose and create the necessary transition from lawn to woodland edge to forest trees.

The long border provides the first step in the transition. Backed up by the rhododendrons, it serves as a natural-looking foreground to the surrounding forest. The two new beds continue the sweeping lines of the long border and form the northern boundary of the cultivated garden, while a crescent-shaped bed to one side of the barn does the same on the eastern front. Turning any of these beds back to lawn would have been an enormous task and therefore counterproductive.

Frustrated by my inability to solve the garden dilemma, I turned to the long-neglected house and began clearing out overstuffed closets, drawers, and bookshelves. Suddenly I felt lighter of heart and better able to cope.

That's when it occurred to me that the same strategy might work out of doors. If I couldn't bring myself to make the garden smaller, surely I could get rid of some things and make it simpler.

However, the gift to be simple was going to be hard-won because there is more to removing large clumps of long-established perennials than meets the eye. Just thinking of the work it would entail plunged me into deeper gloom. At that moment, through the good offices of a friend, Brid Craddock appeared on the scene.

Fresh from the horticultural program at nearby Naugatuck Community College, she brought youth, energy, and a new perspective to the garden. Unlike any of her predecessors, Brid came with a head full of Latin names and theoretical knowledge. She was equipped with a neat canvas bag containing hand tools and a red notebook in which she wrote down everything we did and when we did it.

She sized up the situation at once and concluded that the garden was a lot for two people to handle. While she kept her views to herself, she was obviously relieved when I told her that our first project would be to start simplifying the perennial borders. Made fashionable at the beginning of the twentieth century by British painter and garden designer Gertrude Jekyll, perennial borders are a very labor-intensive form of gardening.

When people think of perennial borders, pictures leap into their minds from the pages of gardening books, magazines, and catalogs. The photographs have been taken at peak bloom and under ideal conditions. Deep borders overflow with a medley of flowers—combinations of annuals and hardy perennials, with a few tender perennials, such as cannas or dahlias, to enrich the mix and extend the season of bloom. Admittedly, borders like this are beautiful to look at but a nightmare to maintain. Their caretakers work nonstop to keep them looking lush but under control.

There are several reasons why mixed flower beds of this type require so much care. First, it's the nature of the beast. Each perennial flowers for a limited time, so the trick is to choose a number of plants with similar flowering schedules for each season and to plan for a succession of bloom from spring through fall. Pulling off such a three-season progression of bloom is a tall order and so is maintaining it.

This is how the season goes in a mixed perennial border. The plants that bloomed in the spring are looking ratty just as the summer bloomers are preparing to do their stuff, while the fall bloomers are rapidly catching up and need to be cut back. So you are cutting down or trying to hide bulb foliage at the same time that you are madly staking peonies before a torrential spring rain bows their heavy flower heads into the mud. Meanwhile, unless you get *Sedum* 'Autumn Joy' and various other tall

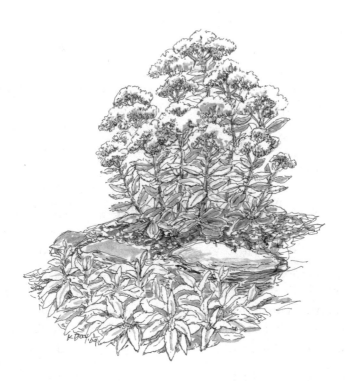

summer bloomers cut back by about a third, the clumps will open up in the middle or get too tall and fall all over their neighbors.

Even easy-to-grow perennials require attention throughout the growing season. For example, daylilies are carefree and un-demanding until midsummer, when they begin to bloom and have to have their spent flowers removed daily, and after they have bloomed, the outer leaves turn brown. The whole clump should then be cut down with pruners to six inches high or the old leaves pulled off by hand.

While other perennials get by with less frequent deadheading and don't need to be cut back, they have other requirements. Trumpet lilies need to be staked to hold up their heavy blos-soms, and tall plants with hollow stems, like meadow rue, also require support. Even big clumps of sturdy rudbeckia look neater surrounded by a girdle of stakes and string.

In addition to needing deadheading and staking, clump-forming perennials benefit from periodic division to maintain their vigor and limit their spread. Performing all these tasks is pleasurable to gardeners but takes time. And dividing overgrown clumps often requires quite a lot of physical effort. In the best of all possible worlds, gardeners would divide their perennials be-fore the clumps got too difficult to handle, but in the real world, overextended gardeners simply do what they can, when they can, if they can.

So that's life in a mixed border. Based on English models, this dense, deceptively casual style of planting was dubbed "care-less rapture" by Lanning Roper, an American expatriate who became one of Britain's most successful garden designers. Fortu-nately, by the time Brid arrived, I had given up "careless rapture" in favor of law and order.

In my perennial borders abundance quickly deteriorates into chaos, so I avoid most self-sowing annuals and tender peren-nials. Even so, reducing the workload was going to mean hard decisions and sacrifice. But once I had help, I decided to begin by removing some of the daylilies.

Brid was the perfect partner in this endeavor because she was not as sentimental as I am about the genus *Hemerocallis*. My affair with daylilies began in 1961 with my very first cultivars and has endured unabated. I still have more than a hundred different cultivars. And despite the fact that some are inferior to others, I love them all. However, they monopolize my time for the entire month of July.

Instead of deadheading every morning, I "break bloom" in the evening, snapping off each blossom while it is still fresh and beautiful. The problem is that at the height of the season breaking bloom can take up to two hours. Usually it is a joy. At sunset, the perfume of the Asiatic lilies, which flower at the same time as the daylilies, begins to drift over the garden. Working my way around the borders is like swimming through alternating currents of cool, refreshing air and scented waves of seductive tropical warmth. By the time I've finished it's nearly dark, and the bats have arrived for the evening mosquito hunt.

I treasure this peaceful time with the daylilies, but if I miss an evening or two, the whole garden looks a mess. So with Brid patiently waiting for me to make up my mind, I hardened my heart and began discarding any daylily with poor foliage. As we worked our way around the garden, I became more and more ruthless. If a cultivar didn't measure up to the late W. R. Munson Jr.'s description of "a good garden daylily," out it went.

Bill Munson, acknowledged dean of daylily hybridizers until his death in 2005, told me once in an interview that his goal was to breed "healthy, happy plants that develop into nice, symmetrical, rounded clumps with good-looking foliage and numerous flowers on strong scapes." *Scape* is the technical name of the daylily's leafless stalk. I added one more criterion, a high bud count—the greater the number of buds to a scape, the more flowers there will be.

However, flowers are not the only consideration in a border. As Brid and I continued our study of the perennials, we began to develop a standard of good garden behavior for each one. Attractive foliage topped the list of desirable attributes. Perennials have a limited season of bloom, but their leaves—for better or for worse—remain for the rest of the growing season.

We gave the highest marks for good foliage to the following: sedums, ornamental grasses, blue star (*Amsonia*), anise hyssop (*Agastache*), calamint (*Calamintha nepeta* subsp. *nepeta*), lily turf (*Liriope*), *Iris pallida*, bowman's root (*Veronicastrum virginicum*), false aster (*Kalimeris pinnatifida*), and blue false indigo (*Baptisia australis*). The leaves of these perennials are an asset in the garden before and even after the plant has flowered.

We found another group only slightly less presentable: catmint (*Nepeta*), white, asterlike *Boltonia,* Siberian iris (*Iris sibirica*), large-leaved lamb's ears (*Stachys byzantina* 'Helene von Stein'), and threadleaf coreopsis (*Coreopsis verticillata*) 'Zagreb'. We did not include the paler yellow, more delicate relation to 'Zagreb', 'Moonbeam', because 'Moonbeam' is apt to die suddenly and inexplicably.

Of all the hardy perennials I have grown, *Sedum* 'Autumn Joy' represents the gold standard in terms of both foliage and flower.

The fleshy blue-green leaves of 'Autumn Joy' are perfection at every stage, from the little rosettes of early spring to the leafy eighteen-inch domes in June to the budded stems in July that look like loose heads of broccoli. These become the flat, fuzzy flower heads, pink in August, turning deep rose-red in September, and finally russet in October.

An inventory of the plants remaining in my streamlined perennial borders is revealing. Instead of a great variety of different genera, there are only a few for each season, not counting the early-season tulips and daffodils. Spring-flowering perennials include eastern bluestar (*Amsonia tabernaemontana*), peonies, Siberian irises, and an old-fashioned bearded iris, probably *Iris pallida*.

I am no longer a fan of the modern bearded irises, which I once lusted after, because borers always wreak havoc with their foliage, chewing the edges of the leaves and coating them with slime. While the plants rarely die, they look so awful that you wish they would. The species *Iris pallida* is a different story. Mine came with the house forty-eight years ago and can still be found in other old gardens. I recently saw it for sale in Williamsburg, Virginia, where the historic gardens contain only plants available in colonial times.

This old iris can be easily identified by its bloomy blue-green leaves, which stand at attention throughout the season and are

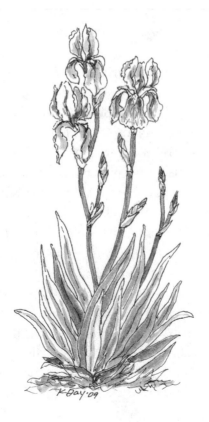

seldom ruined by borers. The three-foot flower stalks bear five or six modest blue-violet flowers that have a delicious scent. And after the brief flowering season in May, the foliage usually remains handsome all season.

Naturally, daylilies survived the purge of midsummer bloomers, but I still have too many so the winnowing-out process continues. A few clumps of blue globe thistle (*Echinops ritro* 'Taplow Blue') serve as a contrast in color and shape to the warm-hued daylilies, but the globe thistles need staking and the leaves and stems have to be cut to the ground after flowering. While they have been spared so far because I love the cool steel-blue color of the prickly, spherical flowers, they face an uncertain future. Plump lavender-blue flower spikes of indestructible anise hyssop (*Agastache* 'Blue Fortune') also provide a contrast to daylilies and are less trouble.

In addition to *Sedum* 'Autumn Joy', other fall favorites that have good foliage and require minimum care include the grasses, lily turf (*Liriope muscari* 'Variegata'), *Boltonia asteroides* 'Snowbank', and *Amsonia tabernaemontana*, the leaves of which turn the loveliest pure yellow. One aster has proved a winner over the years, *Aster* 'Raydon's Favorite', with masses of almost-blue daisy flowers resting on a network of stiffly branched stems and small, coarse, dark green leaves. It blooms at the end of October.

The dried plumes and leaves of the grasses, the flower heads and stems of *Sedum* 'Autumn Joy', and the skeletons of calamint and kalimeris offer their services even during the winter. Once thoroughly dry, they hold up well for most of the winter, unless a freak snowstorm fells them prematurely.

If you have perennial beds that need streamlining and don't know where to begin, the way Brid and I went about it might help you. We started with the daylilies because I already knew that I had too many of them. Next we eliminated some of the plants that always needed staking, like the lovely but ever floppy balloon flowers. We saved one that has unique blue-streaked white blossoms. But we got rid of the last modern bearded iris, one ironically named 'Allegience', which I had loved enough to keep for years. With regret, I parted with what was left of tall *Nepeta* ×*faassenii* 'Souvenir d'Andre Chaudron' because the voles ate more of it every year.

For the last two years, Erica Carroll has been helping me in the garden, and we are continuing the process of elimination that Brid and I started. To my surprise, instead of feeling bereft I feel better. Apparently the remaining plants do too, because the garden as a whole actually looks better.

✤ GLEANINGS ✤

✤ Taking a hard look at perennial borders

When you begin to look for ways to simplify your gardening life, look first at your sunny perennial borders. In my garden, the square footage devoted to flowering perennials demands more time and energy than the rest of the acre and a half under cultivation. The greater the variety of perennials you grow, the more work your border will entail. Some are more carefree than others, but each one demands *something*—staking, deadheading, cutting back, or division—either to ensure good flower production or to restrain its spread.

✤ Biting the bullet

The choice of what to keep and what to part with is highly personal. But if one genus or species monopolizes your time and dominates your garden, think about reducing its number. While daylilies remain my all-time favorite summer-flowering perennials and have many virtues, I simply had too many.

A standard of good behavior

I have worked out a standard of behavior for perennials. In order to remain in my garden, a perennial must be truly perennial and return faithfully every year.

It must be healthy and exhibit the fortitude to endure dry summers without supplemental watering and cold winters without additional mulching, other than the remains of mulch put down in the spring.

It must have superior, or at least good, foliage. Good foliage is attractive for most of the season, which means that some browning of old leaves can be expected after flowering, but cutting it down should not be mandatory. Superior foliage makes an all-season contribution to the beauty of the garden. Think *Sedum* 'Autumn Joy'.

A well-behaved perennial must maintain a tidy habit—no flopping or sprawling. It must remain within reasonable bounds—no overtaking of neighbors or shading them out.

It must not offer an invitation to predators, pests, or diseases. If you have a problem with deer in your neighborhood, you will, alas, have a problem with a great many desirable perennials and bulbs. Among their favorites are tulips, daylilies, Asiatic lilies, and hostas, but the list is much longer.

Dealing with deer

I finally put in a deer fence, but vigilant friends with no fencing report success with repellent sprays and recommend switching brands every couple of months.

Under pressure, deer will eat almost anything, but there are plants that seem relatively deer-resistant. A few, like ferns and grasses, appear truly deerproof. Strongly scented foliage and furry foliage also afford some protection.

Many nurseries offer lists of deer-resistant plants, usually with the caveat that there is no such thing as a completely deerproof plant. Deer are known to avoid daffodils and hellebores, both of which are poisonous, but an enzyme in their stomachs permits them to eat other poisonous plants, like mountain laurel (*Kalmia latifolia*), which would kill cows or sheep.

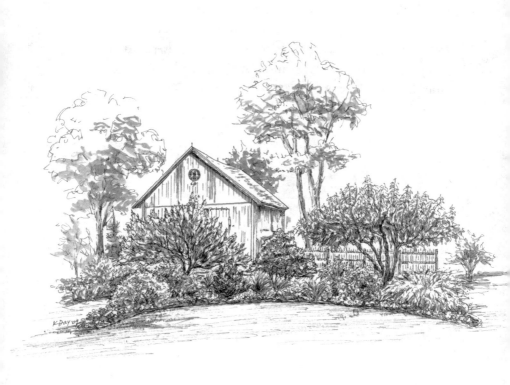

3

A Step Toward Simplicity:
Substituting Shrubs for Perennials

IT WOULD HAVE BEEN far harder to part with so many day-lilies had I not taken this opportunity to plant shrubs in their stead. The perennial borders were the culmination of many years of thought and work, which paid off in waves of color playing across them as seasonal perennials bloomed and subsided, bloomed and subsided, like the Northern Lights. In July, day-lilies were the mainstay of this pyrotechnical display, and to give up any of them saddened me. However, even before 2000 I knew it would be prudent to interrupt that flow of color with a few shrubs. Shrubs need pruning only once or twice a year, instead of the regular deadheading and frequent division required by daylilies and many other perennials.

Years ago, I added a variegated red twig dogwood (*Cornus alba* 'Argenteomarginata') to the long border. Ever since, the dogwood's light grayish green leaves with prominent cream-colored edges have brought light to the back of the border as effectively as a flowering shrub in full bloom. The foliage lasts all season, and maintenance is minimal. Every few years, when the oldest stems lose their dark red color, they get cut to the ground to make room for the younger, brighter stems.

A dwarf Alberta spruce (*Picea glauca* var. *albertiana* 'Conica') joined the dogwood in 2000, followed by a narrow, upright ar-borvitae (*Thuja occidentalis* 'Emerald'). In exchange for the gold, orange, and yellow daylilies that they replaced, the conifers offer year-round color. And the trade-off has improved the bed. The strong conical forms of the conifers create a more interesting skyline and contribute a bit of much-needed geometry. The day-lilies were all about the same texture and similar heights.

More daylilies gave way to the tall vase shape and striking bronze foliage of an eastern ninebark (*Physocarpus opulifolius* 'Diabolo'), which surprised me with small but abundant pink flower heads, a charming contrast against the dark foliage. The ninebark joined a butterfly bush (*Buddleja davidii* 'Pink Delight'), which has an unusually compact habit and gray-green leaves. Fortunately the lavender-pink flowers bloom after the daylilies, which are salmon-pink.

By the time I began working on the newer beds, I already felt the need for more geometry in the garden, and matching dwarf Alberta spruces flanked by clumps of fountain grass (*Pennisetum alopecuroides*) were among the first plants in the ground. The cones of the spruce, balanced by the mounds of fountain grass, held down the ends of the two beds and framed the opening between them. The woody centerpiece of one of the beds is a golden black locust (*Robinia pseudoacacia* 'Frisia') that I gave Martin in 1995. At that time, 'Frisia' was a bit taller than I am, an enchant-

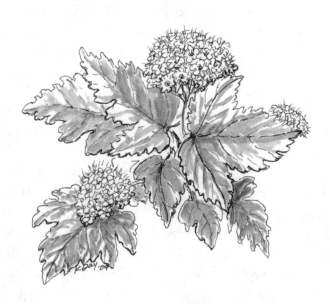

ing little tree with a mop of brilliant yellow-green leaves. Today, it's a tall, narrow tree—perhaps twenty feet high—and rather rangy in habit but still bright and beautiful.

I've grown any number of shrubs over the years. In fact, an island bed on the upper lawn has been one of my most successful efforts. Like everything else in the garden, it has been through many a sea change since 1983, when I planted a dwarf Alberta spruce, a golden false cypress (*Chamaecyparis pisifera* 'Filifera Aurea Nana'), and three blue junipers together. On impulse, I later added a little flowering cherry (*Prunus* 'Hally Jolivette'). To complete this pleasing picture, Elizabeth MacDonald, an artist friend, made us a wonderful blue ceramic ball for the bed.

The blue ball and the cherry shared the spotlight until one year, after flowering gloriously in the spring, the cherry quietly died. For a time the remaining shrubs worked well together, but as the evergreens grew, the blue ball seemed to shrink. Then under cover of a heavy snow, voles stripped the bark from all three junipers, leaving only two of the original shrubs—the spruce and the false cypress. But with the addition this year of two new prostrate blue spruces (*Picea pungens* 'Glauca Procumbens'), the island bed has come into its own again.

Meanwhile, the blue ball has found a new home in the crescent bed. It has come to rest next to a contrasting golden spiraea (*Spiraea thunbergii* 'Ogon'), which has fine, narrow leaves and small white spring flowers. And the spiraea can be sheared to keep it good scale with the ball.

The moral of this story is that shrubs, too, are subject to change, but at a slower rate than perennials, and woody plants are infinitely less trouble. No bed has ever looked better for longer with less work than the island bed. So by 2004, I felt that the time had come to tackle a real shrub border. And in the fall, with Brid's enthusiastic help, I began an ambitious overhaul of the crescent bed.

There were already a couple of large shrubs at the back of the bed. A shapely sapphireberry (*Symplocos paniculata*), probably twelve to fifteen years old, occupied the north corner with a spread of twelve feet. It came from the family home of Netta Lockwood, whom I met only twice but will never forget. Her own garden was the work of a true artist. The charms of the sapphireberry were further enhanced by the person who gave it to me, Robin Zitter, a lovely young woman who was Netta's gardener.

The sapphireberry has proved to be an absolutely trouble-free small tree with shiny dark green leaves that are smothered in May with panicles of small white flowers. While it needs a mate for good cross-pollination, even my lone specimen produces a small crop of lapis lazuli blue berries. The color is beautiful but the birds make short work of the fruits.

A seven-son flower (*Heptacodium miconioides*) stood opposite the sapphireberry, along with the golden spiraea 'Ogon' and *Spiraea japonica* 'Anthony Waterer', which has green leaves. The rest of the crescent was filled with daylilies—recent cultivars from hybridizing friends, some of Gregory Piotrowski's best new ones,

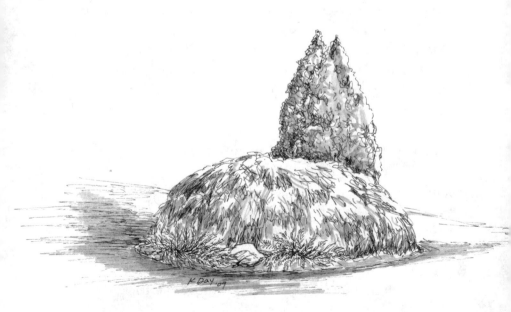

and scores of others. But when it came time to break bloom, my heart sank at the thought of them all. So Brid and I set to with a will.

Homes were found for the daylilies, favorites in my own garden and the others with delighted friends. While a great many were sacrificed to make room for the shrubs, there are still too many left! So the process of simplifying goes on. Meanwhile, Brid and I had planted a linden viburnum (*Viburnum dilatatum* 'Asian Beauty'), two compact oakleaf hydrangeas (*Hydrangea quercifolia* 'Sike's Dwarf'), another golden spiraea (*Spiraea japonica* 'Gold Mound') to match 'Ogon', and a compact weigela (*Weigela florida* 'Nana Variegata').

By the spring of 2006, I realized that the weigela—which was supposed to be "nana," meaning dwarf—was a great deal more robust than I thought it would be and had to be moved before it got any bigger. The rest of the additions seemed to be in pretty good scale, but I am eyeing the hydrangeas nervously. Four feet high is not my idea of dwarf. They are supposed to top out at three feet. But you live and learn—forever when it comes to gardening!

The hydrangeas notwithstanding, the crescent bed looked lovely this spring. It has taken four years for the viburnum to become the beauty it is today, and worth the wait for flat-topped clusters of creamy-white flowers to completely cover the shrub. So far, other than the weigela that needed moving, the shrubs and small trees have required little care.

The seven-son flower needs hard pruning once a year, and the saphireberry a little light pruning, preferably in the winter. The spiraeas are sheared after flowering and again later in the summer. And this spring, I trimmed a few inches off the viburnum, but compared to the endless grooming of the long border and beds A and B, the crescent bed could now be considered low maintenance, which should tell you something about the difference between shrubs and perennials. It certainly impresses me.

✣ GLEANINGS ✣

✤ Why shrubs?

Shrubs afford more value for less work. Some rarely need pruning. I never touch the dwarf Alberta spruces unless a twig or branch loses its needles and dies. Most shrubs suitable for a border are compact varieties and need pruning only once or twice a year.

Shrubs supply strong structural forms—cones, globes, mounds, and other solid shapes—to break up the softness of blossom and to add different heights to the undulating skyline of a border.

Conifers and other evergreen shrubs offer year-round color, while deciduous shrubs with red, purple, gold, or variegated foliage give season-long color. Shrubs like the red and yellow twig dogwoods (*Cornus alba* cultivars and *Cornus sericea* 'Silver and Gold') have colorful stems in the winter and attractive variegated foliage during the summer. Berried shrubs, like native winterberry (*Ilex verticillata*), have red, orange, or yellow berries, favored by many birds. And beautyberry (*Callicarpa bodinieri* 'Profusion') sports clusters of small bright violet berries.

✤ Do your research

It is more difficult to move a shrub than a perennial so you need to be more careful in your selections. If, like me, you buy perennials on impulse, take a little more trouble with shrubs.

Spend time at nurseries, botanical gardens, and the gardens of friends and ask questions like "How long have you had this plant?" and "How often do you have to prune it?"

Consult reference books. Michael A. Dirr's *Manual of Woody Landscape Plants* (Stipes Publishing, originally published in 1975) has been reprinted and revised six times, most recently in 2009. It is still the best of the best.

For conifers, go online and order a copy—new or used—of Adrian Bloom's *Gardening with Conifers*, originally published by Firefly Books in 2002 and in its third printing. The photographs by his youngest son, Richard, are magnificent and show conifers at different ages, stages, and times of year. Bloom is a renowned British plantsman, conifer authority, and creator of a famous garden in Bressingham, Norfolk, England.

❋ Be suspicious of sizes given in nursery catalogs

Even granting the fact that my garden is older than many, the present height and spread of the shrubs greatly exceeds estimates in otherwise reliable nursery catalogs and much gardening literature.

For the same reason, beware of dwarf varieties, especially those that are smaller versions of shrubs and trees that eventually become large plants. Try to find out at least approximate sizes in five years, ten years, fifteen years. I no longer need to worry too much beyond that, but it is information that might once have been helpful.

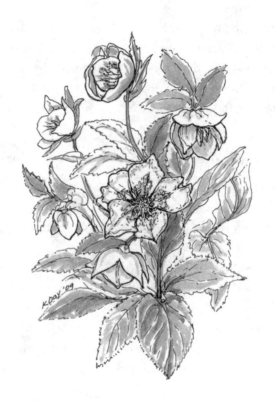

4

Minimum Care:
Appreciating the Shady Border

IT HAS BEEN five years since Brid and I revamped the crescent bed, and I'm glad we started work on it when we did. I've already had five years of pleasure from it even though the conversion from flower bed to shrub border is still incomplete. I thought it needed an evergreen and last year added a lovely little false cypress (*Chamaecyparis obtusa* 'Nana Gracilis'). So far, the shrub border has been a success and much less demanding than any of the perennial borders.

The truth of the matter is that with the possible exception of a rose garden, nothing is more laborious than a sunny perennial border. But a shady border is a completely different story. Mine runs along the stone wall under maples at the edge of the woodland garden. More than a hundred feet long and from ten to fifteen feet wide, it has received no care yet this spring. And it still doesn't look too bad—weeds, yes, where the mulch is thin, but I'm not surprised. We haven't mulched it in three years.

Plants in the shady border that tolerate this level of inattention without resentment include goat's beard (*Aruncus dioicus*) and black snakeroot (*Cimicifuga racemosa*), both six-footers at the back of the border; a few 'Royal Standard' hostas; and in front of them hellebores, brunnera, and corydalis, all enthusiastic self-sowers. In a sunny border I would dread their fecundity, but here seedlings of these plants are most welcome. They fill in among the taller perennials like a ground cover and discourage weeds. More and more, this has become my kind of garden and by comparison with the sunny borders, almost effortless.

Shade is a fact of gardening life in many parts of the world. Wherever rainfall is adequate, trees are nature's chosen ground cover, so it is inevitable that old gardens like mine become shadier as the trees mature. For a time and at great expense, it might be possible to keep the shade at bay, but eventually nature prevails. So I've decided to relax and enjoy it. Besides, what's not to love about a garden that looks attractive from May until November with a minimum of care?

Sun lovers, whose showy flowers are their chief claim to fame, usually require deadheading or other services, while shade-tolerant perennials need little attention and boast handsome foliage that remains a decorative presence in the garden all season. Some, like the hellebores, offer the best of both worlds—picture-perfect foliage for the summer garden and really stunning spring flowers.

My appreciation of the shade and its gardening potential is nothing new. Being surrounded by old maples, my garden has always been shady around the edges, but it is much more so now than when we bought the property. And as shade continues to advance across the hillside behind the long border, I rejoice because there is less and less to do.

In the darkest, driest corner beneath a pair of old maples, ferns, several species of barrenwort (*Epimedium*), and pretty, delicate-looking *Vancouveria hexandra* thrive despite the lack of light and moisture. There is nothing to do here except weed the path once a year, resurface it with pine bark or shredded hardwood mulch, and in the spring, rake out a few leaves around the edges. During the summer, I return periodically to pull weeds that have popped up in the meantime, but there usually aren't many. In the absence of direct sunlight, weeds are easily discouraged by a two-inch layer of mulch.

Under the large maple just behind the long border, hostas, ferns, wild ginger, and Solomon's seal have been growing happily for thirty years with practically no care. In very dry weather they look unhappy, but like a lot of shade-tolerant plants they manage to withstand temporary adversity with aplomb. I have a theory about this. In the wild, shade-tolerant plants generally make their home on the forest floor and are therefore used to low light conditions, root competition, and in southern New England, dry, rocky soil.

That's why many of my favorite perennials for shade are Connecticut natives and other plants indigenous to eastern North America. These sturdy survivors include a quartet of highly desirable native ferns—Christmas fern (*Polystichum acrostichoides*), maidenhair fern (*Adiantum pedatum*), interrupted fern (*Osmunda claytoniana*), and cinnamon fern *(Osmunda cinnamonea)*; wild ginger (*Asarum canadense*); Solomon's seal (*Polygonatum biflorum*); foam flower (*Tiarella cordifolia*); and two species of phlox, *Phlox divaricata* and *Phlox stolonifera*. Of the flowering plants, most are spring bloomers. They get plenty of sun when they need it to flower—before the trees leaf out.

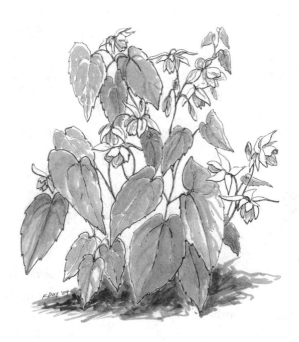

While giving in to nature and growing natives exclusively might make shade gardening even easier, I'm no purist. I also grow and enjoy shade-tolerant plants from many other parts of the world. The Christmas rose (*Helleborus niger*) hails from the wooded mountain slopes of Switzerland, southern Germany, Austria, and northern Italy. The stinking hellebore (*H. foetidus*) is also from Europe, and the Lenten rose (*H. orientalis*) from northern Greece, Turkey, and the Caucasus. No shade garden should be without these hellebores.

First to bloom, the Christmas rose is perhaps the most beautiful for the purity of its large white flowers, nodding above dark green palmate leaves. The stinking hellebore follows with mops of smaller chartreuse blossoms at the apex of tall, sturdy stems and narrow, very dark green foliage. The unflattering common name refers to the smell of the flowers and leaves, but unless you purposely crush them it takes a good imagination and a better nose to detect any odor.

The Lenten rose, a favorite of hybridizers, is completely scentless. Its lovely flowers, similar to those of the Christmas rose, now come in a luscious shade of crushed raspberry, dusky plum-purple, and tints of pale pink. The whites can be pure and unadorned or embellished with purple freckles. The leaves of the Lenten rose are palmate, like the other two species, but broad, shiny, and a fresh medium green.

Familiarity with hostas can only breed admiration. Among foliage plants, they are the best of the best. Most are native to Japan, with a few species occurring in China and Korea. While there are only twenty or so species, hybridizers have created innumerable cultivars, and their magnificent leaves come in every size imaginable from minute to enormous. The color range is equally broad, spanning every tint, shade, and hue from golden yellow to powder blue. The golden hostas light up the shade like shafts of sunlight penetrating the forest canopy, and the blues rest the eye and soothe the spirit.

Besides the solid-color hostas, many cultivars boast interesting patterns of variegation. The green-and-white ones are among my favorites because they look so fresh and crisp. The patterns include green leaves splashed in the center with milky white, predominantly green leaves with tidy white rims, and green with broad brushstrokes of white around the edges.

Stalwart, beautiful, long-lived, and getting better by the year, hostas perform flawlessly—until they begin to flower. Regrettably, the scapes begin to bloom from the bottom up, like the blossoms of foxgloves. But unlike the spent flowers of foxgloves, which fall off and don't ruin the appearance of the whole spire, shriveled hosta blossoms cling doggedly to the scape and spoil the look of the whole inflorescence. Many gardeners cut them as soon as they appear, forgoing the flowers entirely. Cutting down the scapes after flowering is a nuisance, but otherwise hostas are perfect perennials—things of beauty, a joy almost forever, and a great boon to shade gardeners.

If I could have only two perennials for the many shady places in my garden, they would be hostas and ferns. Few pairings are

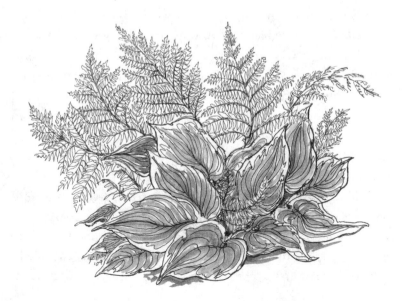

so ideal. While their cultural needs are a perfect match, their shapes and forms create a dramatic contrast in pattern and texture. The mighty leaves of the big hostas, radiating outward from the crown and overlapping in giant mounds, provide the perfect foil for graceful, upright ferns like the native cinnamon fern and the interrupted fern. The simple outlines of the hosta foliage set off the delicate texture and intricate fish-bone pattern of the ferns.

Although most of the ferns in my garden are native to this area and are used in informal shade borders, the fern-hosta combination suits even a formal garden, because both players are essentially sleek, refined plants. I have used this combination repeatedly on the slope behind the long border, adding an edging of wild ginger rescued years ago from the clutches of poison ivy along our road.

Of all the small filler plants for shade, I love best and could not do without two species of *Corydalis* or common fumitory: yellow (*C. lutea*) and white (*C. ochroleuca*). They cover their foot-high clumps of finely cut blue-green foliage with thousands of little tubular flowers from March to November.

In the large semiwild area under the Chinese chestnut tree, *Corydalis ochroleuca* has its own way, self-sowing with abandon. Here it mingles with another prolific self-sower, heartleaf brunnera (*Brunnera macrophylla*). Similar in behavior and culture but highly contrasting in texture and form, they are another ideal couple. The bugloss has large, rough, heart-shaped leaves and in the early spring puts forth sprays of small brilliant blue forget-me-not flowers. The lacy fumitory, with its little white flowers, wanders about between them.

A few years ago, to give the irregularly shaped bed a semblance of order I added an edging of bushy, indestructible cranesbill (*Geranium macrorrhizum*), which has handsome leaves and pink flowers in June. Hemmed in by the geraniums, the patchwork of self-sowers carpets the ground at the feet of rhododendrons and a *Magnolia virginiana*, a native tree with a smattering of lemon-scented white flowers that also appear in June. Here in the north, it will eventually reach about twenty feet. Except for pulling out jewel weed and keeping an eye peeled for vagrant strands of poison ivy, I give this bed no other care.

Like many of the shady areas in the garden, the semiwild bed was never turned over or prepared in any way. I dug holes, amended the soil with compost, put in the plants, and covered the ground around them, first with layers of newspaper and then with a 3-inch layer of hardwood mulch. Even mulching is no longer necessary because the tapestry of plants completely covers any exposed soil.

In the fall, leaves from the chestnut and other nearby trees cover up the whole works. Spring cleanup consists of blowing off excess leaves, tidying up, and mulching the edges of the bed. What sunny border would be so easily satisfied?

✣ GLEANINGS ✣

✢ The good news about shade

Shade-tolerant plants are easier to maintain than sun lovers. One of the reasons is that weeds are also sun lovers. In the shade, they become feeble and can be controlled by a layer of mulch.

Also, there are relatively few prima donnas among the shade-tolerant plants. Most are low-key and undemanding, even those with eye-catching flowers. For instance, the flower spikes of astilbe are exceptionally decorative, but after they have bloomed the dried stalks don't look too bad.

❀ Shades of shade

In the Northeast, old gardens feature shrinking areas of sunlight and growing patches of deep shade, usually from large trees with dense canopies. Deep shade describes a substantial reduction of light throughout the day.

Light shade is a desirable condition produced by a group of birch trees or other trees that have small leaves that flutter with the wind and allow light to penetrate their airy canopy.

The ambiguous description "sun to part shade" can mean either shade lovers that can take the gentle morning sun or sun lovers that flower well enough with a full morning of sun and afternoon shade.

❀ For dry shade, consider native plants

Dry shade puts additional stress on garden perennials ill adapted to such conditions, but many native woodlanders are naturally tolerant of both dry soil and low-light conditions.

Wherever climatic conditions are difficult or inhospitable to garden perennials, look to the natural landscape for guidance in choosing plants. Native doesn't mean out-of-control plants with a rumpled appearance. You couldn't ask for more civilized plants than native ferns, Solomon's seal, and wild ginger.

❀ Nonnative shade plants with style and stamina

In addition to the common perennials that appreciate shade, there are nonnative woodland plants with the style and stamina for any shady site. They include European and Asian versions of our own mayapple, wild ginger, and

Solomon's seal: Himalayan mayapple (*Podophyllum emodi*), European ginger (*Asarum europaeum*), and the beautiful variegated Solomon's seal from Japan (*Polygonatum odoratum* 'Variegatum').

Also on the list are the barrenworts (*Epimedium* cultivars), mostly from the Far East; tall Japanese yellow waxbells (*Kirengeshoma palmata*) with flowers at the tips of stems covered with large maplelike leaves; and one of the few grasses that like shade, Japanese forest grass (*Hakonechloa macra* 'Aureola').

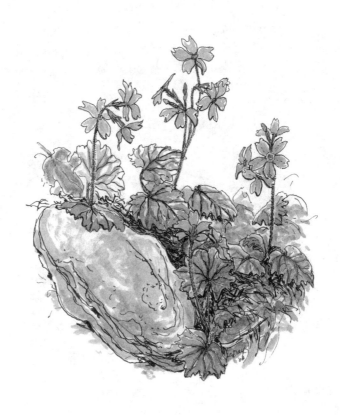

5

Woodland Gardens:
Living in Harmony with the Forest

OF ALL THE SHADE plantings, the woodland garden is the most forgiving and the one dearest to my heart. It reminds me of my homesick English mother and of myself as a child, combining as it does primroses from the countryside she left behind and the New England wildflowers of my youth. At a distance, nothing distinguishes the woodland garden from the state forest. The trees are assorted sizes—a few older trees, young trees, saplings. Some are crowded together or oddly shaped. That's what I love about the woodland garden. It doesn't *look* like a garden. Even the path around the pond is so irregular and narrow that it might have been made by deer.

The woods are my natural habitat. When I was growing up, our house was surrounded by a cluster of struggling farms, their pastures, and hundreds of acres of woodland. For my younger brother and me, all this was our playground. In the winter, we explored the woods for caves and followed animal tracks. In the spring, streams were a great source of interest to Hugh, who looked for good fishing pools while I hunted for wildflowers.

Small wonder that city life never suited either of us and that as adults we figured out ways to live in the out-of-doors—Hugh on a wild mountain slope in Washington state and me in the gentler hills of Connecticut. The woods surrounding my garden are much the same as the woods where Hugh and I played—the same tree species, similar gray, lichen-covered rock outcrops, and small streams that eventually find their way to rivers.

For me gardening in the woods was a natural, and discovering the little stream on our property made it inevitable. Spring is announced every year by the sound of rushing water, echoing back to the house from down by the barn. It is a wonderful sound, wild and free. The temptation to play in the stream was always strong. However, I was still commuting to my teaching job twenty miles away, and summers were spent making perennial beds and pushing back the brush and weeds to uncover the stone walls.

It wasn't until the spring after I left my job that I responded to the siren song of the stream. At that time, there was no actual streambed; the water simply raced downhill from the overflowing swamps above, squeezed through an opening in the stone wall, and emerged in a rush before fanning out among the rocks.

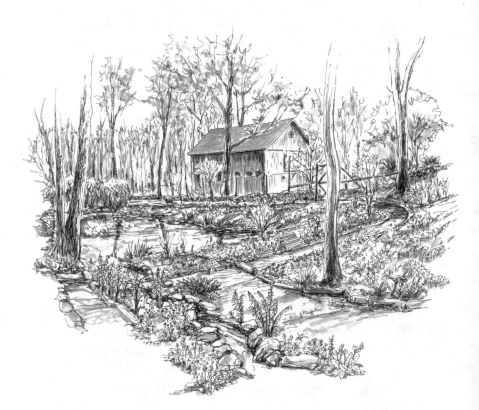

As the land leveled off, little rivulets of water began to wander in a leisurely, aimless way down to the hollow behind the barn.

Our predecessors had tried digging out the hollow to make a swimming hole but abandoned the project when they realized that the water source was winter runoff, not a viable spring. So by the time I began to take a serious interest in the woods, the bottom of the pond was thick with red maple saplings. That summer, a high school boy armed with loppers and a bow saw helped me cut them all down. And I've been playing there ever since.

The fortunes of the woodland garden have ebbed and flowed with the ups and downs in my own life. And for the last four years, that part of the garden has endured almost total neglect. The miracle is that so many of the plants have survived, primroses from the British Isles, Europe, and Japan along with native wildflowers: phlox (*Phlox stolonifera*), marsh marigolds (*Caltha palustris*), violets, Dutchman's breeches (*Dicentra cucullaria*), wood poppies (*Stylophorum diphyllum)*, mayapple (*Podophyllum peltatum*), Virginia bluebells (*Mertensia virginica*), twinleaf (*Jeffersonia diphylla*), bellworts (*Uvularia perfoliata* and *U. grandiflora*), and an abundance of ferns.

In July 2007, a kind volunteer appeared on the scene and helped me remove that year's crop of weeds from along the woodland path. The next spring, an English gardening friend came to stay in March, and we cleared leaves out of the stream and did a bit of raking. But it wasn't until the following spring that I had enough help. Erica Carroll came to me with experience in maintenance, a passion for plants, and a quick, eager mind that absorbed everything. She caught on immediately, did wonders for the perennial borders and for my morale, and even spent a few odd moments weeding in the woods. Otherwise, from spring 2005 until the spring of 2009 the woodland garden was left to fend for itself, and fend it did.

Of course, in the early days, I poured time and energy into

what Martin called my "mud garden." I persuaded the stream to steer the course I set for it in a narrow, rock-lined canal, complete with tiny pools and waterfalls. My next project was to build up the banks—there was absolutely no soil—with alternate layers of leaves, topsoil, and compost. The compost had to be brought in by the bucketful because the opening in the stone wall was too narrow to admit a wheelbarrow. A few years later, I found a wider breach in the wall, and the talented Emile Racenet, a landscaper of many gifts, fashioned a whimsical gate for it out of twisted cedar branches. His pièce de résistance was a primrose flower cut out of a rusted plowshare.

From either gate, the path goes all the way around the pond, then up one side of the stream and down the other. About three hundred feet long and no wider than a deer track, the path re-

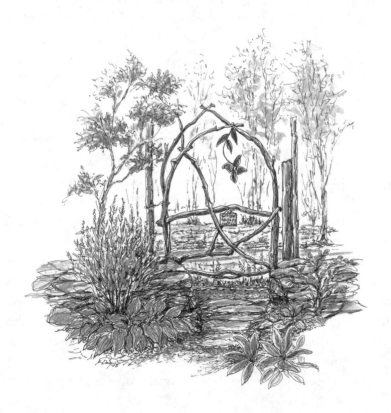

quires approximately fifteen bags of mulch to resurface it once a year. The primroses grow in liberally amended soil along both edges of the path and at one end of the pond. The area covered by the woodland garden is small—one hundred seventy-five feet long and seventy feet wide, with the pond (really a vernal pool) occupying about two-thirds of it.

When I joined what was then called the American Rock Garden Society, I met H. Lincoln Foster and his wife, Laura Louise, always known as Timmy. It was one of the best things that could have happened to the woodland garden and to me. The Fosters were a legend in the gardening world, and Millstream, the garden they created together, was a place of pilgrimage. It remains in my memory the most beautiful woodland garden I have ever seen.

Imagine an entire mountainside covered with acres of mature azaleas and rhododendrons, many of them Linc's own hybrids. Among the broadleaf evergreens, the stream that had once powered the mill wheel bounded noisily down the mountainside between banks covered with Japanese candelabra primroses. And along the narrow, winding footpaths, wildflowers, native and exotic, familiar and unfamiliar, formed great swaths of color. At every turn, there was something wonderful to see—a rare Jack-in-the-pulpit from Japan or an unusual primrose from Russia.

Suffice it to say that Millstream and the Fosters provided inspiration for my woodland garden. They also offered me an education, patiently teaching me plant names and introducing me to *Primula* species I had never heard of—*P. abschasica*, a species from the Caucasus, and *P. kisoana* from the Himalayas and Japan. They told me how to grow primroses and shoveled treasures out of their garden into mine. Thus, for a few years my *Primula* collection was quite extensive.

Sadly, many of the choicer species require better soil, more water, and more care than I could provide. And today, only half a dozen stalwarts remain, three species from Europe and three from Japan. According to the American Primrose Society, these are the easiest to grow for most gardeners in the Northeast.

Even a drop of British blood almost guarantees a love of primroses. Every spring my mother, who was born in Devonshire and grew up on the west coast of England, pined for primroses. Fortunately, her favorite, the common English primrose (*Primula vulgaris*), is one of the survivors in my woodland garden. It has delicate single blossoms of moonlight yellow arising from a clump of crinkled oval leaves. The cowslip (*P. veris*), a rough-and-tumble relation, is another survivor. Cowslips are still going strong, sending up stalks bearing tiny bright yellow blossoms in loose umbels. The oxlip (*P. elatior*), assumed to be a natural cross between the first two, has actually colonized a mossy north-facing bank of the vernal pool. The flower of the oxlip looks like both parents, having the umbellate form of the cowslip and the much larger flowers of the common primrose.

The doughty Japanese species include the tall candelabra primroses (*Primula japonica*) with tiers of outward-facing flowers in shades of pink and red. *Primula kisoana* has lovely scal-

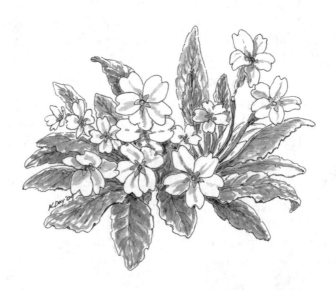

loped leaves, fuzzy six-inch stems, and small clusters of pink flowers, and easy-to-grow *P. sieboldii* produces larger clusters of white, pink, or mauve flowers. This primrose escapes the summer by going dormant.

Make no mistake, most primroses cannot be considered perfect perennials in the Northeast. Mine look just plain awful in the summer, but no one has to see them then, hidden as they are down behind the barn. In a severe drought, even the European species go dormant. It alarmed me the first time it happened, but most of them put out new rosettes of leaves in the fall.

Unfortunately, our summer heat and humidity are anathema to them. And they don't like winters much better, unless snow blankets the ground and stays there until March. Otherwise, even under their natural mulch of fallen leaves many of them heave out of the ground when it freezes and thaws. As the plants are covered up, I don't see them in time, and they lie there with their roots exposed until they die.

In this climate, what primroses really like is snow cover in the winter, and moist soil, rich in organic matter, with good

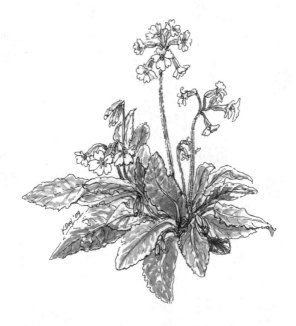

drainage. They would also infinitely prefer light or dappled shade to the dense shade that overtakes my woodland garden by June. But a surprising number hang in there, and I love them for it.

The rest of the plants in the woodland garden are natives that just take it as it comes. So for a really easygoing woodland garden, use only indigenous plants or a mixture of native woodlanders and tough shade-tolerant perennials from other places in the world. Avoid both natives and exotics that require too much care or spread outrageously.

The chief mistake I made in the woodland garden was in not really understanding the habits of some of the native plants I employed. To my cost, I discovered that mayapple has territorial ambitions beyond my wildest dreams and that the self-sowing propensity of the wood poppy boggles the mind. As for including the magnificent ostrich fern (*Matteuccia struthiopteris*), I must have been mad.

In F. Gordon Foster's excellent book *Ferns to Know and Grow* (Timber Press, 1984), the author spells it out very clearly: "Leaves rise from a crown; dense underground runners, extending in all directions, reach out to establish new plants. Restrict planting to large areas or where spreading can be controlled." As a result of my ignorance, ostrich ferns have taken over a large area at one end of the woodland garden, and every year I invite—no, beg—a friend to take as many as she can to cover up a vast, shady bank in her woods.

Ideally, the woodland garden should be weeded and the leaf mulch topped up early in the spring, late in June, and once again sometime before fall, when the weeds in the bottom of the pond have to be cut down with a string trimmer. But if no one gets to it, I'm learning that love *can* be blind.

❧ GLEANINGS ❧

❧ Possibilities in a patch of woods

A woodland garden can be as small and simple as a handful of stepping-stones around a couple of trees and a few
clumps of primroses and native ferns. Or it can be as ex-
pansive and complex as the Fosters' Millstream.

If you are fortunate enough to have at least a buffer
of second-growth forest between your house and a neighbor's, you have the makings of a woodland garden. You
can start by raking a narrow path among the trees, cutting down whatever saplings or understory shrubs are in
the way. Cover the path with a few bags of shredded hardwood mulch or bark.

For shade-tolerant plants to put along your woodland
path, consult this and the previous chapter.

❧ Planting under and among trees

In soil woven through and through with tree roots, the
easiest way to plant is to scrape out pockets between the
roots, amend what soil there is with compost, mound it
up, let it settle, and plant on top of the mound.

In the woodland garden, I used logs to raise the planting area on either side of the path four or five inches and
added a layer of old leaves covered with topsoil laced with
liberal amounts of compost.

✤ Essentials for a woodland garden—soil amendment and mulch

Tree roots are so greedy that it is imperative to improve the soil with moisture-retentive organic matter, like compost, and keep the surface covered with an organic mulch. The protective mulch will preserve moisture and gradually decompose, improving the soil.

Nature mulches in the fall with leaves, but if you disturb the surface layer at planting time, you will have to replace that covering. Water new plants for the first summer.

✤ Ongoing care of a woodland garden

A woodland garden shouldn't need much care. Mulch and water the plants until they fill in. After that, weeding a couple of times a year should be adequate.

I created work years ago by having Martin cut too many trees. Given so much light, weed seeds germinated instantly and took over.

Another mistake was to plant native plants that proved too aggressive for such a small garden. However, the combination I used to combat the weeds—ostrich fern, mayapple, and wood poppy—is perfect for a large woodland garden.

✤ The six easy primroses for woodland gardens

If I have been able to whet your appetite for primroses, here are a few to try. From Europe and the British Isles: *Primula vulgaris*, *P. veris*, and *P. elatior* and their hybrids.

From Asia: *Primula japonica*, which requires constantly moist soil and is perfect for the edge of a real pond or stream. The other two are less particular: *P. sieboldii* and *P. kisoana*.

All six species are hardy in zones 4 to 8. They find hot, dry summers harder to bear than cold winters but appreciate snow cover.

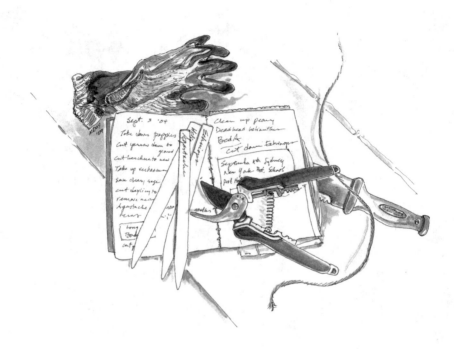

6

Sanity Saver:
Learning to Make Lists

MARTIN USED TO SAY that we were "shot through with luck." And it's true. We had it all—peace, privacy, and each other, an old house in the country and a garden. That's how life was the summer before Martin's death in 2005. We had no idea that he had cancer. It must have been very slow growing, and thankfully there were no symptoms. He felt tired sometimes, which annoyed him but did not surprise either of us. After all, he was eighty-three. As he loved to read and to play with his new computer, being less active didn't bother him much. And he was secretly relieved to have the mowing taken off his hands.

In retrospect, the timing of Brid's arrival during this grace period was another stroke of luck. It gave us time to get to know each other and for Brid to become familiar with the garden. With nothing more urgent on my mind than the garden's future, I was able to focus on the maintenance problem.

Having recently decided to make gardening her career, Brid wanted more hands-on experience. Her background was in graphic design, and she had completed her course work in horticulture. She also had a new garden of her own, which she had planned and planted, and was maintaining with the help of her husband. What she needed was an established garden in which to practice her craft and hone her skills. What I needed was a pair of willing, capable hands. We were a perfect fit.

In the end, she did so much more than mulch, stake, weed, and deadhead; she saved my sanity. Because she was coming to horticulture from the corporate world, organization, multitasking, and setting priorities were second nature to her, while they were utterly foreign to me. My approach to gardening had always been visceral and visual. I didn't want to *think* about it, I just wanted to *do* it, look at it, and figure things out as I went along.

Brid, on the other hand, was a born planner. When I couldn't see the woods for the trees, she gently pushed me to make lists of what we needed to accomplish in the four hours she spent with me every week. She insisted with great tact that we first do a "walkabout."

Out would come the red notebook and around the garden we would go, with a package of large white plastic plant markers in hand. Whichever perennial needed attention, I was to make a note on the stake and stick it into the ground next to the plant. She would do what needed to be done. By the time she left that day, she would have done it.

I attribute much of her efficiency to the list-making habit. It

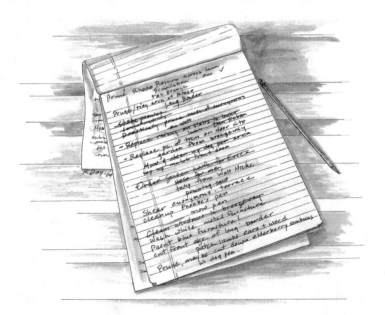

is a technique frequently recommended by self-help books to establish order and reduce stress. Writing something down gets it on paper and off your mind. Heretofore, my list making had consisted of grocery lists and appointments hastily scribbled on the back of an old envelope. But at Brid's urging, I prepared a "to do" list every week before she arrived. We still did the walkabout, but we were able to do it much more quickly and efficiently.

Indeed, the weekly list for Brid proved so helpful that I was open to another idea, the creation of a master list. The object is to include literally everything—tasks both great and small, from clipping a single straggling branch from one of the rhododen drons to mulching the flower beds. What makes this extensive list so valuable is that instead of going outdoors and being so overwhelmed by the enormity of what has to be done, you can choose one thing and actually get it done.

If I'm feeling fainthearted or have only a few minutes, I pick something small like cutting off the offending rhododendron branch. I'm happy because the plant looks better, and I have the added satisfaction of crossing something off the list. Admittedly, compiling it in the first place is a tedious, time-consuming job, but it's well worth the effort. Here is a sampling from last season's master list:

Rake, blow, pick up sticks and twigs on lower lawn
Seed bare patches on upper lawn
Fix damage to driveway retaining wall
Clean up edge in front of forsythia hedge
Prune forsythia hedge
Move forsythia 'Golden Tide' from long border to left of
     driveway
Mend, glue, and nail loose strips of lath, front gate
Cut back variegated weigela
Cut down suckers of *Hamamelis mollis*

Lop tall, upright branch sticking out of *Rhododendron*
 'English Roseum'
Order tarp from Walt Nicke catalog
Edge front of long border
Move *Agastache* 'Golden Jubilee' to bed A
Patch holes in the lamb's ears in front of long border
Divide *Hemerocallis* 'Mini Pearl', bed B

Calling the newer perennial borders bed A and bed B was
another of Brid's bright ideas. It made it quicker and easier to
locate a specific plant requiring her services.

When I perused last year's list for the purpose of writing this
chapter, I was pleasantly surprised by how much had actually
gotten done. I knew from the start that some of the things
wouldn't get done at all and that tasks I deemed important at the
time might not seem so later. For instance, no one ever got
around to raking the twigs and litter off the lower lawn. But
when the lawn was mowed for the first time, the twigs were
chewed up or run over and eventually decomposed anyway.

Last fall, I learned about another kind of list making from
Dan Sieban, the young man who remodeled my kitchen. Home
improvements and repairs had always been Martin's department,
though we worked on big projects together. Now, of course, the
house is my responsibility and part of the overall maintenance
picture. Anyway, the kitchen hadn't been touched in forty-five
years, and a few changes were long overdue. But I did not want
and could not afford to rip everything out and start from scratch.

Instead, Dan began to make the necessary improvements little by little, a few days here, a few days there. In between, he told
me to keep a "punch list" of any small carpentry jobs I needed
doing. Apparently, the term is used in the building trade to de-
scribe the list used to keep track of all the loose-end jobs that
have to be completed before the work is considered finished.

So I began to keep a running list for Dan, for the electrician, and for the plumber on the extra pages at the back of my month-at-a-glance calendar. Plumbers and electricians charge so much for just showing up that you don't want to forget something and have to get them to come back again.

I use the garden punch list in the same way. I make note of jobs that will require either special expertise or additional manpower. For example, in the old days Martin served as resident plumber. Our water supply was never adequate for an irrigation system, but he and I laid PVC pipe out to the various garden beds, and he put in sill cocks so that I could run hoses to newly planted shrubs and perennials. Every fall, Martin disconnected the pipes at the house, and I gathered up the hoses, put them in the cellar, and went around opening the sill cocks to drain out the water. I still do my part, but now I have to call a plumber to disconnect the pipes. A reminder to make that important call should be on the garden punch list, which is much shorter and more specific than the master list.

The biggest job of all in this garden is the mulching, and extra help at the beginning of the season can pay off. Brid proved to me that it was cheaper to buy shredded bark mulch by the yard, have it delivered, and hire an able-bodied young man to put it down than for the two of us to spend all summer hauling three-cubic-foot bags around the garden.

She and I could do the flower beds, which we mulch with leaves. But shredded bark is more effective and lasts longer on the paths and under the apple trees. The downside of the bark mulch is that it is so much heavier, and it took us forever to spread it.

Setting priorities was another of Brid's strengths and my weaknesses. At heart I'm a perfectionist, which I used to think laudable. It isn't. It's laughable to expect perfection in a garden, which never remains static. But I wanted the whole garden to look immaculate. While it never did—nature saw to that—it came close during the nineties. But time marches on. Shrubs and even trees outgrow their positions, and circumstances change. Adjustments must be made, which in a way is what makes gardening so endlessly fascinating.

Anyway, by the time Brid came into my life I was a bit more flexible but still preferred to get one bed completely finished— weeded, mulched, and edged—before going on to the next. However, she pointed out that we would never get around the whole garden that way. It would take too long. Instead, she suggested that we get as many of the beds weeded and mulched as possible and leave the edging until last. And how right she was! Edging as I knew it has gone by the boards anyway.

However, mulching is absolutely essential to maintaining the garden. It virtually eliminates weeding in the flower beds and helps retain moisture in what is otherwise a very dry situation, and eventually the mulch decomposes and improves the quality and texture of the soil. Never since I began using the leaf mulch have I fertilized the flower beds, and the plants have always appeared healthy and happy.

Cutting the edges of garden beds is an expensive luxury. It requires a special crescent-shaped tool or a very sharp spade and a modicum of skill. Every cut must overlap the pervious one to

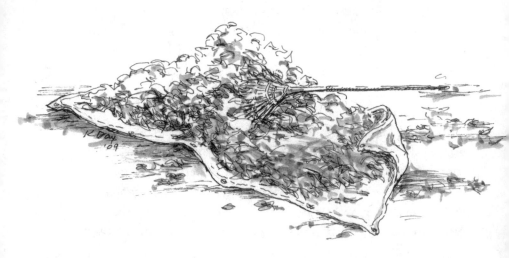

achieve a clean line. Even with two people it takes hours, because the sod has to be removed by hand and carted off to the compost pile. For a straight edge, you need string stretched between two stakes and pulled taut. Curves can be laid out with a hose, which also serves as a guide.

Deata and I were good at edging, and we took the time to do it. One of us would cut the edge, the other dig out the sod, and Ross would come along with the wheelbarrow and pick up after us. But it got harder and harder to get around all the beds, and in the end we cut only the front edges. Brid and I couldn't even manage that except on rare occasions. Her time and my energy were too limited.

Today, a new lightweight edging tool that has an almost knife-sharp blade makes cutting sod easier, but it still has to be removed. For the same reason, a beefy little electric Edge Hog proved unsuccessful. So now, except when we are expecting garden visitors, the edges of the beds are weeded by hand and the shaggy grass kept down with the string trimmer.

For the three years that Brid was with me, the entire garden looked presentable because she knew how to hit the high spots and keep us up to speed. The first year, she took notes of what we did and when. The following year she was able to consult the red notebook and tell me that it was time to cut back the purple smoke bush or that next week we should stake the grasses. Grasses have to be staked while they can still be coaxed up through the grid of wire that will support them later in the season.

Within the first hour that Brid spent in the garden, I knew that she was exactly what I needed. Martin's assessment, after the three of us had lunched together, was "good value," a very English way of saying the same thing. I also knew from that day that this ideal arrangement would be short lived. A teenage daughter would soon be looking at colleges, and when that happened Brid would have to get a properly paid full-time job.

The time came much too soon. Brid tided me over the hard

summer after Martin's death. Her cheerful, upbeat presence and sturdy work ethic got us through the season. Reluctant to leave me without help for the following year, she put me in touch with Peggy Weaver, another wonderful gardener and a dear person. But her schedule was even tighter than Brid's. Peggy had two other jobs and three children still at home. Although she gamely stuck with me through the fall, we both knew that I needed more time than she could give me. So the search for help began anew.

❧ GLEANINGS ❧

❧ List making

It's not an original idea, but when you feel overwhelmed by all the things that cry out to be done in the garden, making a list can be useful.

Keep the daily list short because you probably have too many other obligations already.

If you are lucky enough to have help in the garden, a list for your helper will save you time and therefore money. Both will be better spent.

❧ The master list

This idea came from my college roommate. She suggested compiling a master list of absolutely everything that needed attention in the garden, no matter how large or small. While the master list became staggering in length, a year later I was amazed to see how many items had been checked off.

This is how the master list works. Let's say that you have only thirty minutes to spend in the garden. Without that list, I would end up frittering the time away trying to decide where to begin. With the master list, I pick something quick and easy and actually get it done. And there is the added satisfaction of crossing it off the list.

In addition to the master list, I also keep a short ongoing list of jobs that require expert help, such fixing a leak in my watering system or solving deer fencing problems. This list is kept on a page of my month-at-a-glance calendar because forgetting to make those calls can have dire consequences.

✤ Establishing priorities

In a large garden, it is important to practice a sort of horticultural triage. Some things are essential; others are not. While I dislike the verb *prioritize* as much as I dislike doing it, I'm getting better at it, and list making has helped.

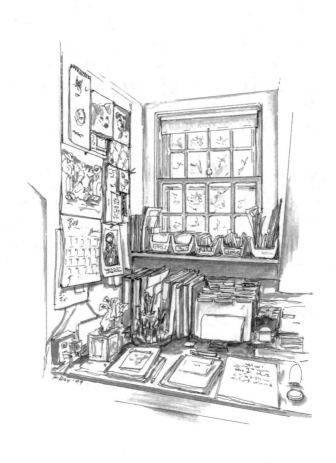

7

Juggler's Dilemma:
Searching for Help

EVERYONE WHO HAS ever worked in my garden, from Lou to Brid to Peggy and now the invaluable Erica, has come to me through a friend or by word of mouth. However, if you are looking for help for the first time, you need to begin by casting a wide net. It's not enough just to ask gardening friends. Friends who don't garden and are looking for someone themselves are often your best bet.

That's how I found the admirable Casey, a college student in need of summer employment. He was working for a friend who was too busy to garden. She knew that I had been looking for someone, too, and when she didn't need Casey for a full day, she called to see if I had a couple of hours of work for him. I did. Erica and I were happy to have him, because we were expecting a group of garden visitors the next day.

If you need to look farther afield than your neighborhood, try the nearest community college or branch of your state university's cooperative extension service or any institution that holds gardening classes. Botanical gardens and arboreta offer programs in horticulture and can be a valuable resource. If all else fails, there is still word of mouth. But it doesn't happen spontaneously; you have to get the word out by initiating conversations with everyone you meet wherever you find yourself—at the post office, at the checkout counter of the market, or in the waiting room of your dentist's office. Sooner or later, someone will have a friend or relation who is interested in gardening and looking for work.

Getting the right kind of help is something else again, because every site and every garden is different. Also, there are as many ways to garden as there are gardeners. What is important to me may be less so to you or have nothing to do with what you need. But I'm happiest if whoever helps me in the garden appreciates the natural beauty of its setting and realizes that the garden is most successful where the hand of the gardener is least in evidence.

Peggy loved the garden, and gardening with her was a joy. We worked well in tandem, because we were as alike as two peas. In the spring, we lavished attention on the shade plantings behind the long border. The path among the rhododendrons, refreshed with a new layer of wood chips, looked more inviting than ever and there wasn't a weed anywhere. But we lost sight of the big picture, and the big picture is what makes this garden. Peggy and I were too much alike. It's better to have someone whose gardening style complements yours rather than duplicates it.

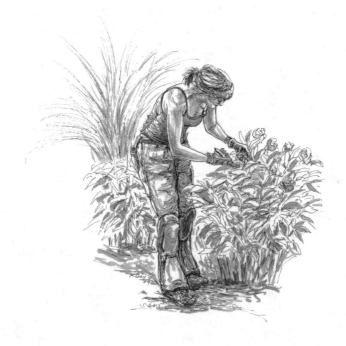

In the end, of course, you're lucky if you find someone who will put up with you and help you keep the garden from going to wrack and ruin. But to make any arrangement work, you have to be clear about what you want and understand what is possible. The question is, given the time, energy, and expertise that you bring to the partnership, how many hours a week will it take to achieve a level of maintenance that satisfies you and is appropriate to your budget?

There is no easy answer, because all you have to go on is previous experience and an educated guess. And because circumstances change, the answer depends to some extent on the season. Some years you have more time and energy than others. But it goes without saying that as you get older, your energy diminishes. In calculating time, I have always erred on the side of expecting too much and underestimating how long it takes to achieve the desired result. However, the last few years have taught me to be more reasonable and more realistic.

For the foreseeable future, given what I can still do myself, my guess is that I will need one capable, energetic person for five or six hours a week. That's what I can realistically afford. And that is not really enough for the big jobs, such as cleaning up and mulching in the spring and dealing with the leaves in the fall. During her all-too-brief tenure, Brid dragooned Harvey, her patient, good-natured husband, into helping us with these tasks. And this year for spring cleanup, Erica brought a young man with her.

Martin and I had always done the fall cleanup with whomever was helping in the garden. And we had a good system. The two younger members of the team raked and blew the leaves into piles; Martin would shred them with the Gravely tractor by tilting the deck and dropping it down on the pile. Then either the raker or the blower would vacuum up the shredded leaves with the second tractor and dump them behind the barn.

If we kept up with it every week during October, leaf removal wasn't hard, but it was time-consuming. Having a landscape crew do the work cost too much, as I discovered the year Martin was in an auto accident that put him out of commission for the fall. While nothing can ever replace Martin and his beloved old Gravely, Erica and I managed last fall without calling in reinforcements.

Like most gardens, mine is at its most demanding at the end of one season and the beginning of the next. In between, the ongoing work in the flower beds has already been substantially reduced by giving away perennials and substituting compact shrubs. But there are still three massive hedges to shear, a lot of pruning to do, and deer fencing to keep in running order. Martin used to check it twice a year and repair it if necessary. But it hadn't been tested regularly since his death, and last September I found telltale deer droppings in the woodland garden.

An urgent call to a friend who is a landscape designer produced the name of an outfit that deals in specialty agricultural

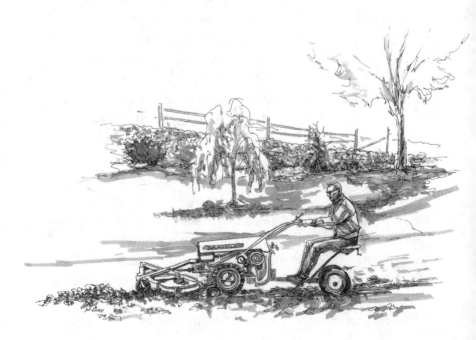

products, including deer fencing. Fortunately, their response was quick; the problem was traced to the charger and easily solved. Martin always bought a backup charger when he replaced the old one, so I had one on hand. Purchasing a new charger is now an item on the punch list.

I was lucky to have an in-house handyman, but unless you do or are knowledgeable and experienced yourself, you would be well advised to hire someone for electrical problems. And you have to budget for this eventuality. Another expense that I was never fully aware of is the servicing and repair of power equipment, like the garden tractor, leaf blower, electric hedge trimmers, and other electric or gasoline-powered tools. That was always Martin's department, so I didn't know the real cost of maintaining a garden like ours. I'm a wiser woman now.

Like it or not, you need to be aware of these hidden expenses in order to figure out what you can afford in terms of helping hands in the flower beds. Simplifying them was a good start. Now that they demand less of our time, Erica and I can give the woodland garden at least a lick and a promise, fit in some pruning, and do the leaves in the fall. The only additional expense is for the strong back to help us with mulching in the spring.

I know that an exhaustive discussion of garden maintenance is the last thing gardeners want to read, but it really is the crux of the matter, and I'm afraid there is more. No matter how much we love our gardens, they are only part of our lives. Everyone of my vintage—my gardening friends, the people I meet at garden clubs—is struggling to balance the many opposing demands on our hearts and minds, our time, energies, and pocketbooks. Any sort of crisis wreaks havoc with that precarious equilibrium.

My garden is inseparable from the rest of my life, which included when Martin was alive the house, two vehicles, the reigning Jack Russell terrier, family, friends, and visitors from England. Responsibility for this ménage was a joint effort, each of us doing what we did best. Martin took care of house maintenance and repairs, paid the bills, dealt with the finances, and latterly did the shopping. I cooked, cleaned the house, kept up the garden, coped with dog training and trips to the vet, wrote articles and books, and traveled around giving garden talks. It all worked relatively smoothly and fit together. But without Martin, nothing seemed to work.

Now I do the things for which I have no aptitude and in which heretofore I had taken no interest, and I am not finding it easy. House, garden, dog, family, friends, and my writing have all been shortchanged. Even the car is presently in dire need of service. I suspect that this is familiar territory for everyone of a certain age. But a bright spot named Anne Harrigan has recently appeared on my horizon and made life a lot easier.

In the spring of 2007, three years after Martin's death, I was asked to open the garden to a group from the Federated Garden Clubs of Connecticut. I had been saying no much more often than yes to such requests, but it was to be a special occasion for a small group, and the person who contacted me was so nice and so persuasive that I couldn't refuse.

The women who came that day were warm, appreciative, and kind, and I found myself talking about the difficulties of keeping the place up and my sadness at having to let weeds take over the woodland garden. Later, as the group was leaving, Anne stopped and said, "I'll help you weed your woodland garden." She called the next week to tell me that she had Thursday mornings free, and she has been coming ever since.

There is no job description for what Anne does, but having been a secretary for forty years, she is extremely orderly and efficient. She has helped me sort out my desk and files, deal with the mail, and move the potted plants upstairs for the winter, and she waters them when I forget. In the last few months, she has also taken over some of Martin's chores, like picking up office supplies at Staples, mailing packages, and doing the shopping.

In five short words borrowed from William Wordsworth, she has made "Oh, the difference to me!"

As you try to balance all the demands in your life, keep in mind my experience with Anne. It was a complete surprise to discover that it wasn't the garden that was weighing so heavily in the balance, it was the minutiae of life as an older single woman. The devil was in the details.

You, too, may find that what you need is someone to free you from some of the myriad small household tasks so that you can spend more time in the garden. Even if you don't know what you need and feel completely overwhelmed, there is someone out there who can help you. You just have to keep looking, keep talking to people, and keep an open mind.

Don't underestimate the charms of the older gardener. One friend of mine, no longer as spry as she once was but still a superb gardener, barters with a young horticulturist, trading treasures from the garden in return for labor. I have recently gotten to know a young man who is in the throes of becoming a passionate gardener, and he offered to help me after coming to a program I did at a local nursery. Terence Farrell and his family have been a great addition to my life and a godsend in the garden.

Quite apart from the pleasure of their company, I have been helped by Terence and the twins, six-year-old Ryan and Caitlin, to plant a hedge of *Sedum* 'Autumn Joy', divide dozens of daylilies, shear the long forsythia hedge, and prune huge old junipers. They even pitched in with the leaves one cold, windy day last fall. And I don't know where I would have been without them when Erica was out for a month last summer with a shoulder injury. The moral of this story is: never say no to any offer of help.

Older people sometimes feel that age has diminished their worth, but one of the lovely things about gardening is that in the eyes of young gardeners, age and experience confer status. When I was in my forties, a mere child in the gardening world, I worshiped at the feet of older members of the North American Rock Garden Society—Linc Foster, Harold Epstein, Dick Redfield, Geoffrey Charlesworth, and Norman Singer.

In return for my wholehearted admiration, they gave generously of their time, which becomes increasingly precious with age; their knowledge, which was deep and broad; and their plants, which came from the far corners of the earth. It's my turn now. When I send Terence home with daylilies or visit his garden, I think of these dear people. They, too, had everyday lives and struggled with the same balancing act that we all do, but their gardens kept them going, just as yours and mine will keep us going.

❧ GLEANINGS ❧

❦ Determine what kind of help you need

If you can afford it, have big one-shot jobs like transporting, delivering, and spreading several yards of bulk mulch done by a landscaper or a handyman with a truck.

For ongoing help with perennial borders and pruning shrubs, you probably need someone you can teach or someone who already has some experience.

❦ How and where to find gardening help

First, ask fellow gardeners. On my behalf, Rita Buchanan, whom you will meet in Chapter 10, asked her friend Robert Herman, a faculty member at Naugatuck Valley Community College, if any of his horticulture students would be interested in working in my garden. And Brid raised her hand.

Inquire about horticulture programs at high schools

with vocational agriculture programs and at local community colleges. You will find information online and in the phone book.

Contact the cooperative extension service offices in your state about local Master Gardener programs. These programs provide volunteers with training in horticulture. In return, the volunteers make themselves available to answer gardening questions at local extension service offices and spend a minimum of thirty hours on community gardening projects. Gardeners who have completed the program and fulfilled their obligations often start their own gardening businesses and post notices on the extension service's bulletin board.

Public gardens, botanical gardens, and arboreta that offer continuing education programs are possible sources of help.

❧ Once you have found help

When you have found someone, you must be clear about what you want done and realistic in your expectations.

Given what you can do yourself and the number of hours of paid help you can afford, what is reasonable and possible?

Remember that you may care more about your garden than anything else except your family, but the person working for you may also have a family and other interests and can only do so much.

❧ Anticipate the possibility of needing extra seasonal help

Spring cleanup is always the most labor intensive in my garden, because winter storms rain down twigs and branches and damage the old trees. For the name of a licensed arborist, ask friends and consult the sources already mentioned.

Early spring or late fall is also the time to get power equipment serviced. Call the power equipment place where you bought your tractor; they usually pick up and deliver, but it takes time, so plan ahead.

Fall cleanup can also require either extra help if you do it yourself, or a landscape service.

❧ The juggler's dilemma

Modern life puts great demands on young and old alike, making every day a juggling act. As you get older, it becomes harder to keep all the balls in the air.

So stop for a few minutes, sit quietly in the garden, and figure out what weighs on you most. I discovered that it wasn't managing the garden. It was managing the rest of my rather chaotic life.

If you love to garden yourself and are fairly able-bodied, you may not need gardening help. Instead, you may need a smart, reliable person who you like and trust to come for a couple of hours a week to sort mail without throwing out the credit card bill and to make appointments for you. Whatever you need, there is someone out there who can help. If you belong to any organizations or a church, ask there and keep asking.

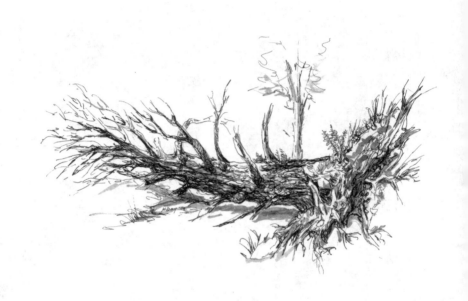

8

Lessons from the Garden:
Accepting Imperfection

OF ALL THE LESSONS that gardening has taught me, the hardest to digest inwardly has been the acceptance of imperfection. As a young teacher, I was profoundly irritated by a student who never managed to finish an assignment. She wrote in longhand and would recopy an entire paper if she made the tiniest mistake. I know now why I found her perfectionism so maddening: I'm like that myself. But when it comes to the garden, I'm gradually learning to go with the flow and to appreciate the glorious moments for what they are, brief and beautiful. Shakespeare's contemporary Ben Jonson well understood that "in short measures life may perfect be." Perfection in life and in the garden depends on a counterpoise too fragile to maintain because time is always moving forward.

My garden was carved out of abandoned farmland in the early stages of returning to its wooded state. All around me, the miles of stone walls threading their way through the state forest attest to the fact that the landscape continues to evolve. These walls once enclosed hayfields and cow pastures. In making the garden, I have only delayed the natural progression to woodland.

Even mature woodland continues to change, albeit at a more measured pace than a garden of herbaceous perennials, but steadily and inexorably. Just beyond the garden walls, trees that have completed their life cycle now lean at odd angles, their fall broken by neighboring trees. No one takes down the dead trees with a chain saw. Eventually their own weight does the job, and when that happens a hole opens up in the leafy canopy. For the first time in years, light and moisture find their way to the forest floor, and long dormant tree seeds germinate. The fallen tree begins to decompose and becomes food for the seedlings of the next generation. Ongoing life is nature's reason for tolerating imbalance, imperfection, and impermanence.

Absorbing this lesson has been good for me and for the garden. Now instead of slavishly raking every leaf out from under the shrubs in the fall, I do the opposite and blow as many as possible back under them. This heavy layer of leaves protects shallow-rooted plants like the rhododendrons from extreme temperature changes and eventually breaks down and provides nutrients for the plants.

The same laissez-faire policy can also benefit lawns. Grass is, after all, a plant. It can tolerate regular shearing but only if the amount removed does not exceed a third of its height. And instead of being vacuumed up or blown away, the clippings should remain on the lawn to revitalize the shorn grass plants.

In the spring, don't wait to start mowing until the lawn becomes a hayfield. Begin when the grass is four to six inches high and set the mower blades so that you don't cut off more than an inch of the top growth. If you use a lawn service, whoever mows your lawn will be happy, because conservative mowing may mean more frequent mowing at the beginning of the season. There is, of course, an alternative. Learn to live with longer grass until the growth rate slows down in June. In the summer, it's better to leave the grass on the long side anyway. Mowing too close inhibits root development, weakens the grass plants, and in extreme cases kills them. During periods of heat and drought, cool weather grasses react to the stress by going dormant, and the shorter the grass is cut, the quicker the lawn will turn brown.

When Martin was young, he and his sisters played tennis in their garden on a fine-textured, weed-free grass court, but summers in Yorkshire bear little resemblance to summers in Connecticut. Grasses that flourish in the cool, damp north of England would soon succumb to drought, heat, and humidity in southern New England.

Martin was quite content with our lawn, which is made up of mowed field grasses, clover, and other weeds. We used to patch bald spots and occasionally seed over thin places with whatever seed mix we found at the local Agway. Neither of us cared enough about lawn to do research into different kinds of grass seed. I was much too interested in making perennial beds, and Martin in tinkering with the power equipment. To each his own. Thus, the mowing fell to him.

Every week or ten days, he would dutifully mount the tractor and cut the grass. But during the dog days of August, he didn't stir from his air-conditioned office upstairs. The lawn was left to its own devices. As the days cooled off and became shorter and the rain came, the grass began to perk up. And by the end of September, it looked quite respectable again. So when August rolls around and the days are long and hot, take a tip from my spouse. Relax in the shade and forget about mowing. You'll have plenty of opportunity later, because grass does most of its growing in the fall and spring.

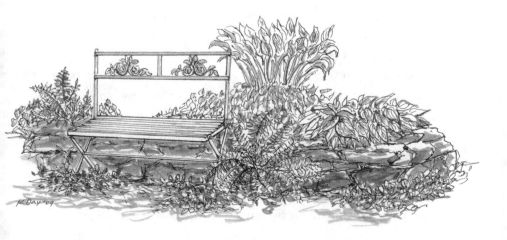

While I am more or less resigned to this approach to lawn care, honesty compels me to admit that in my heart of hearts, I'm envious of people with smooth, green, weed-free lawns. There is nothing more flattering to a perennial border. But that kind of lawn takes more time, effort, money, and water than I have at my disposal and requires heroic measures I would not want to employ. The application of chemical fertilizers and weed controls would endanger not only the ground water but also my own health and welfare and that of the small dog with whom I share the lawn and garden. So I have arrived at a compromise.

This coming spring, I am going to have about a third of the upper lawn slit seeded. The water table should be high enough in April to permit watering as necessary. And in May, I'm going try corn gluten, a high-nitrogen organic fertilizer. When I've watered it in, I'll sit back and hope for the best. Summer care of the lawn is in the hands of a local landscape company, which is willing to mow no lower than three inches and not at all during droughts. In the fall, they resume their regular weekly schedule.

If I were ten years younger and had more time, I might go to greater lengths to improve the grass and do research on the right grasses for this climate. But for now, experimenting with corn gluten is all I'm prepared to do. I recently heard about it in an excellent lecture entitled "Lawn Care with the Environment in Mind" by Joann Gruttadaurio, a professor of horticulture at Cornell. And I might still contact the Cornell University Cooperative Extension Office to discuss better turf management and learn about the latest improved grass varieties. According to Professor Gruttadaurio, the type of grass seed you use can make a big difference in the health and appearance of your lawn.

Besides letting your lawn alone when it's hot and dry and avoiding the use of fertilizers and weed killers on it, you can save yourself a lot of work by taking the same approach to your garden. It's gratifying when labor-saving garden practices are easier on the gardener and at the same time kinder to the planet.

I haven't sprayed with anything but water laced with a few drops of dish detergent for at least thirty years, and the plants don't look much worse than when I was using lethal chemicals. According to my 1962 garden diary, I was advised by a reputable nursery to combat an insect problem on border phlox with a combination of pesticides that would curl the hair of any conscientious gardener of today.

While we may still be a long way from sustainable gardening, we have certainly made progress since the sixties. Even in England, where gardening techniques have remained the same for generations, new ideas are challenging old.

In the September 2007 issue of *The Garden*, the magazine published by the Royal Horticultural Society, Matthew Wilson wrote about a new approach to gardening. The most telling rev-

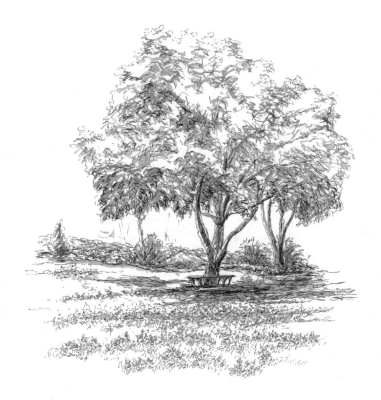

elation was his own epiphany. Having graduated from horticultural college fifteen years earlier, he wrote: "I feel that the biggest lesson I've learned since leaving college is that whatever we do in our gardens, nature will always win out, so far better to be in tune with it than deploy prescriptive, outmoded practices." I hope this theme is beginning to sound familiar.

Elsewhere Mr. Wilson asks, "Does it really matter if our lawns have a few daisies and our roses a few aphids? Rather than going straight into battle, is it not better to retune our aesthetic antennae and garden more sympathetically both with nature and our changing climate?" I believe that American gardeners are ahead of their British counterparts in employing more environmentally friendly practices, such as encouraging beneficial insects. A few aphids might attract ladybugs, whose larvae feed on these small soft-bodied pests, while chemical pesticides kill insects both good and bad.

Mr. Wilson also reports that the time-honored practice of double digging for perennial borders, which I read about in English gardening books of my day and actually did in my first flower bed, is no longer recommended. Instead, a new approach to soil management has proved better for the garden and for the gardener's back.

Your garden soil can be improved substantially by the surface application of organic matter, like compost or the leaves used in my garden. Allowed to break down naturally, it works just as well as double digging and isn't nearly as arduous. So put your best efforts into mulching and let the worms and microbes do the rest. I have been doing it for years, thanks to Louise Marston, a disciple of the late Ruth Stout.

Lou, whom I met through my gardening mentors Helen and Johnny Gill, knew a thing or two about soil because she made her own. She lived and gardened on her daughter's property in Bethel, Connecticut. It was a cliff of bare rock with a driveway like a goat track. I will never forget my first visit. I parked on the road below and walked up.

On a narrow shelf of ground at the base of the cliff sat a pile of rotted hay and another pile of steaming cow manure, the main ingredients of the soil that Lou created. She began by making little stone walls in front of the cliff and layering first hay, then manure; more hay, then soil scraped up in the surrounding woods, and finally a mulch of leaves, also procured from the woods. In the beds, this concoction had already become the kind of soil that gardeners dream about.

Roses hid the base of the cliff and campanula festooned the homemade retaining walls. Between them, yellow and white bearded iris held their elegant blossoms high above billows of *Geranium* 'Johnson's Blue' and tussocks of pink dianthus. All this—and more—was possible because a few years earlier Lou had read Ruth Stout's classic *How to Have a Green Thumb Without an Aching Back.*

Mrs. Stout began practicing and touting the benefits of compost and mulch in the 1950s. When I met Mrs. Stout some years

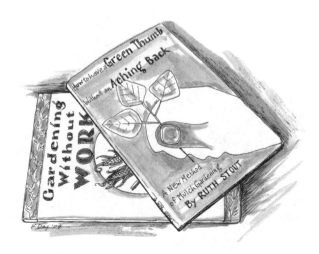

later, she was in her nineties and still going strong. Martin and I had the privilege of driving her home after a party and saw her garden. You couldn't miss it. Enclosed by four high walls of chain-link fencing, it had once been a tennis court. Now it looked suspiciously like a vast compost pile, which is not surprising.

Mrs. Stout had a healthy respect for the leftover vegetables and fruit rinds that most people call garbage. "What is repellent about these things?" she demands in her book. "They were quite inoffensive before you tossed them into the garbage pail. Why do they change character the minute they lose their individuality and become garbage?" She hadn't a qualm about tucking garbage under both vegetables and the flowering plants in her garden, and it was as lush as a jungle. In effect, she grew her garden in the same fresh organic matter that I put on the compost pile, only she saved herself that extra step.

Ruth Stout gardened and lectured well into vigorous old age and died a happy woman, partly because she had long ago mastered the art of cooperating with nature and going with the flow.

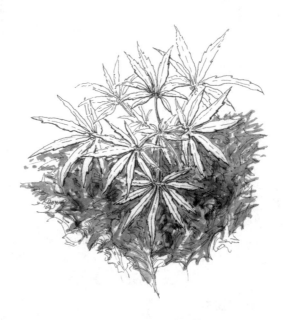

❧ GLEANINGS ❧

❧ Nature will take its course

Life is perfect only rarely and briefly, and gardens are the same. Living things are always in a state of becoming. A seed becomes a mature plant, which enjoys a brief prime, ages, dies, and becomes compost to nurture a new generation. As that is how nature works, our best hope of a simpler way to garden lies in learning to go with the flow.

❧ Accepting imperfection

Nature does not clean up every dead leaf in the fall, and gardeners don't have to either. Dead leaves left under shrubs serve as a mulch, which eventually breaks down and contributes nutrients to the soil.

Nor do gardeners need to rake or blow grass clippings off the lawn. If the mowing is done at an appropriate height, the clippings will sink to the ground and eventually revitalize the grass plants.

We need a whole new attitude toward lawn. I'm coming around to the view that if it's short and green, it's lawn. It would be nice to have a weedless greensward, but the price is too high in terms of manpower, chemicals, fertilizers, and just plain water.

❧ Lawn care

Don't mow too close at any time of year, but especially when the weather is hot and dry. Shorn grass plants are stressed grass plants.

During a drought, it is better not to mow at all. Many grasses go dormant in extreme heat but soon revive with the arrival of shorter days, cooler nights, and more rain. In the meantime, learn to live with a less-than-perfect lawn.

Don't expect perfect flowers every year either. Some years, insect damage is considerable; other seasons, it's light. Either way, don't spray. Insecticides kill insect friends and foes alike and pose a risk to your health and that of your pets.

❧ The beauty of mulch and compost

Covering the soil with a layer of organic mulch is the greatest favor you can do yourself and your garden. Initially it is a laborious task, but it saves hours of weeding.

More important, organic mulch benefits plants by keeping the soil cool in hot weather and retaining moisture. By decomposing and becoming compost, mulch ultimately becomes organic fertilizer.

The late Ruth Stout, author, lecturer, and maven of mulch, wrote a book that modern gardeners should read for its common sense and rollicking good humor. Long out of print, *How to Have a Green Thumb Without an Aching Back* is worth searching for online and at book sales.

Mrs. Stout put a grin on the solemn face of organic gardening. Having found a simpler way to garden back in the fifties, she continued to garden that way until her death at the age of ninety-six in 1980.

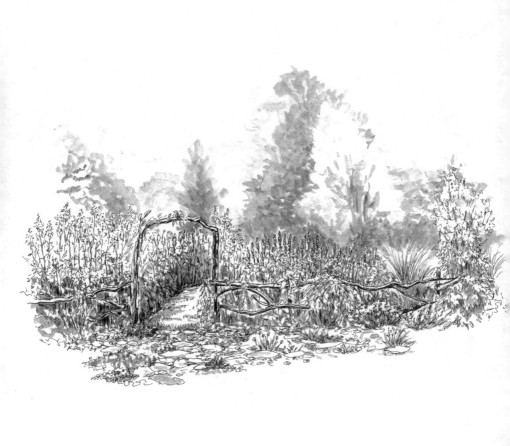

9

From Lawn to Meadow: Learning from Experience

WHEN MARTIN AND I drove Ruth Stout home that day, I don't recall there being any lawn around her small, shingled brown house. I doubt that Mrs. Stout would have approved of turfgrass. Too much upkeep for too little reward. She clearly preferred more interesting and productive plants, like flowers and vegetables. Nor is she alone. My friend Mary Stambaugh has being divesting herself of lawn ever since I met her more than thirty years ago.

When she and her late husband, Harold Ley, bought the property at the top of the highest ridge in our hilly town, three acres were devoted to lawn. To preserve a spectacular view of the Litchfield Hills to the north, their predecessors had cut down trees and spread out a vast carpet of green turf that rolled gently down the hill and into the wooded valley. This vista had always been maintained by regular mowing. Mary, however, had other plans for her hillside.

Before long, artfully arranged groups of rocks, dwarf shrubs, and alpine plants began to eat into the pristine green slope. Meanwhile, lawn on the south side of the house was undergoing a similar transformation. By 1981, it was unrecognizable. What had once been immaculately groomed grass had all but disappeared under a sloping mass of rocky debris. As more rocks and gravel arrived by the truckload, Mary's bewildered husband found himself sympathizing with the farmers who had spent the best part of a century clearing away the rocks from this land. But in his wife's talented hands, the scree became a magical place of miniature mountains and valleys with rivers of poppies running through them.

Among the rocks that her friend Karl Grieshaber, former curator of the rock garden at the New York Botanical Garden, had so skillfully placed, dwarf conifers created high points and accents. In the early days, alpine treasures nestled at their feet, enjoying the bright sun and sharp drainage. But over the years, many of the small plants have with Mary's blessing given way to large patches of thyme and other ground covers. The conifers, no longer dwarf, now rule the rock garden, and the only maintenance required is weeding the gravel paths.

Back in the early 1980s, Mary had only begun her crusade to eliminate lawn, and with it gasoline-powered equipment. Her next project was to turn the vast greensward to the north into a flower-filled meadow. It proved to be a daunting task, one that

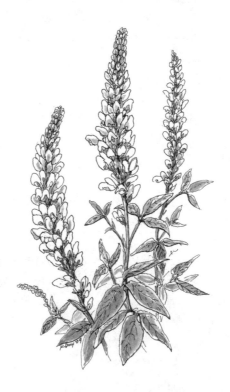

has taken many years and demanded not only her best efforts but also those of the people who worked with her, chiefly Rob Cuchetto and Laura Evans. Along the way, there have been steps forward and steps backward. However, the first step was easy enough—too easy, as it turned out. She just let the grass grow. But the effect was not what she had in mind. So she marked off large sections of the hillside with string and had Rob plow them up.

She sowed seed from a regionally correct "meadow in a can" mixture, only to have the seed swept away during a heavy rainstorm. She tried again, this time with some success. The native grasses and coreopsis survived, along with Carolina lupine (*Thermopsis villosa*) grown from seed that came from her grandfather's garden in Cincinnati, Ohio. The individual seeds were large enough and heavy enough to hold their own against the elements.

Next, Mary changed tactics and started perennial wildflower seed under lights in her basement. To ensure survival of the seedlings, she grew them on until they were stalwart enough to tolerate life in the wild. This proved a much better technique, and she has managed to establish large colonies of flowering perennials that have naturalized and are now to a large extent self-supporting.

Weeds and unwanted woody plants, like the invasive *Rosa multiflora*, still do find their way into the meadow and have to be grubbed out by hand, and over the years she and Rob have dug up "tons" of overenthusiastic native goldenrod. She admits, "A meadow like this doesn't just grow. It has been a maintenance-ridden project but visually a great success and such fun. I love waiting for things to come up and bloom—something different in every season."

Among the most successful perennials in her meadow is the yellow Carolina lupine from her grandfather. This lovely native plant has spread by its underground stems, sending up dozens and dozens of tall lupinelike flowers in late June. Another winner is closely related blue false indigo (*Baptisia australis*), which blooms earlier. I gave Mary a few clumps of a native sunflower, *Helianthus mollis*, with large yellow daisy flowers and gray-green foliage the texture of suede. These sunflowers have really taken off and in their turn light up the field in July. Purple coneflowers bloom at the same time. Nowadays, there are hybrids in sunset shades of orange, yellow, white, and pink, but Mary's plants bear the mauve-pink rays and prickly orange centers of the species *Echinacea purpurea.*

In August, goldenrod and purple New England asters create a beautiful color contrast and look wonderful with tall clumps of pink Joe Pye weed (*Eupatorium maculatum*) and purple New York ironweed (*Vernonia noveboracensis*). These taller native plants shoot up among the shorter wildflowers, reaching heights of six feet or more. And the show of yellow and purple continues well into the fall with later blooming asters and goldenrods.

Rather than a meadow, Mary calls her flowering hillside "a gardener's interpretation of a meadow" because she has included suitable nonnatives such as tall, airy purple meadow rue (*Thalictrum rochebrunianum*) from Japan and orange tiger lilies (*Lilium lancifolium*), also Asian in origin. The design of the meadow garden is simple. A wide, grassy path flows through the middle, carving its way down the hill through walls of tall grasses and wildflowers. It invites wandering and also provides access to different sections of the meadow for purposes of management.

While this wonderful garden feature cannot be considered really low-maintenance, it requires less regular attention than the lawn it replaced. Instead of thousands of identical grass plants that had to be mowed weekly, a colorful array of largely native grasses and perennials gets by with a once-a-year mowing. Although maintenance is still an issue, this garden is easy on the environment, requiring neither fertilizer, pesticides, nor irrigation. And it hums, buzzes, and chirps with the vital life of birds and insects, which give Mary joy and a sense of connection with her land.

Kim and David Proctor's version of a meadow also replaces lawn, but they took a different approach, one in keeping with their hectic work schedules and family life. Kim, whose drawings add so much to this book, has always juggled multiple jobs—the lot of most artists and designers—while David, a hardworking sales rep, has a long daily commute. Both love gardening and so do their children.

Son Ross shares a magnificent bonsai collection with his mother and works at a wholesale nursery. Daughter Lee is in her second year at Penn State, studying floriculture. She and her father plant an enchanted and enchanting vegetable and cutting garden every year around the little shed that David built. With so much on their plates, the senior Proctors decided to simplify their lives by getting rid of unused lawn.

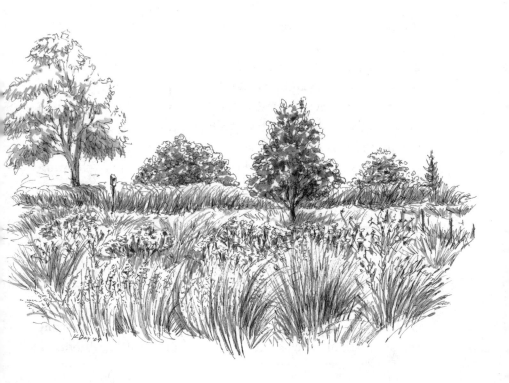

As Kim explains, "The kids are away most of the time now, so there are no more soccer games and there is a lot of lawn that we don't use for anything. It just seemed silly for David to spend so much time mowing. So we cut a diagonal across a big long rectangle of lawn and let the grass on one side grow." By mid-summer, the Proctors were surprised and delighted to discover that their lawn was a diverse mixture of grassy plants and native wildflowers.

Long-discouraged asters and yarrows found themselves free to grow, bloom, and go to seed. Different grasses, sedges, and even a few rushes from the nearby wetlands had a chance to mature, proving that not all grassy plants are the same. To explain the difference between grasses, sedges, and rushes, Kim quotes a useful little poem. Her version appeared in the catalog of Oliver Nurseries, the Connecticut nursery where she grew up and worked for many years. I've since discovered that other slightly different versions abound in the world of horticulture. But here is Kim's: "Sedges have edges / Rushes are round / And grasses are hollow all the way to the ground."

As the season progressed, differences in the heights and textures of the grasses and grasslike plants began to emerge, adding variety to the new meadow, which covers about an eighth to a quarter of an acre. The most strongly growing and prominent among the grasses is meadow fescue, a fairly coarse grass with wide blades and pretty seed heads that appear late in the summer. Sedge, with its long, narrow, glossy blades forms graceful masses two and a half to three feet high at the edge of the wetlands area. The presence of a few clumps of soft rush (*Juncus effusus*) was a complete surprise. Kim describes it as "a sweet grassy plant with absolutely round stems about two feet high."

"It was fun," she says, "to watch and see what happened over the summer. It changed quickly, as various shapes, forms, and colors came and went. In a short time, it went through amazing transformations. David and I would pull out our Adirondack chairs and drag them to the edge of the meadow, where we would eat lunch and watch the birds."

The Proctors' old farmhouse sits well away from the main road in the middle of their property. At the back David mows to the woodland edge, and on the south their new meadow blends into neighboring wetlands, where moisture-loving native shrubs like winterberry (*Ilex verticillata*), silky dogwood (*Cornus amomum*), and gray dogwood (*Cornus racemosa*) create a suitable and attractive background. Thus, the meeting of garden and landscape is seamless because many of the same plants appear in both places.

The Proctors' low-key, environmentally friendly approach to meadow making began in the spring of 2008. They simply took a hoe and a steel rake and scratched up three-by-six-foot areas of the meadow. They didn't dig out the sod, but they managed

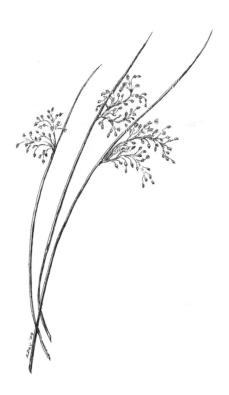

to expose enough soil to give a foothold to wildflower seed. Then they ordered a mix from Ernst Conservation Seeds, a company specializing in native and naturalized plants of eastern North America. Having sown the seed, they waited to see what would happen.

Twice during the growing season, Kim and David went through their new meadow and hand pulled a few of the bigger weeds. Otherwise there was nothing to do except enjoy the sprinkling of brightly colored annuals—mostly coreopsis and cosmos—that grew from the wildflower mix. The annuals made themselves at home among the resident perennials and grasses and quickly attracted approving flocks of birds, especially finches, which came to feast on the cosmos seeds. It remains to be seen whether the annual wildflowers will maintain themselves by self-sowing or be crowded out by the grasses and perennials. But on the whole, the Proctors are well pleased with their meadow.

At the end of the season, David succeeded in cutting it down with the lawn tractor set at its highest setting, but it was slow going, and another time he would consider renting a brush cutter for the day. Already he has more ambitious plans for next year. That's the trouble with gardening. It is a chronic complaint that can't be cured, but as you age it must be managed.

✤ GLEANINGS ✤

✤ A gardener's interpretation of a meadow

Mary Stambaugh has a wonderful three-acre wildflower meadow. She calls it "a gardener's interpretation of a meadow" because the hand of the gardener is evident in the tides of different seasonal flowers that surge across the hillside.

The sheer variety of flowering plants this veteran gardener has grown and planted far exceeds what would normally appear in a northeastern meadow. While the effect is lovely beyond words, making this meadow required a great deal of time and effort.

Mary succeeded in establishing wildflowers in her meadow only by first growing the seed under lights in her basement, planting the seedlings out when they were large enough to hold their own, and then weeding around them until they became established.

✤ The trouble with meadows in a can

The seed for wildflowers and grasses may come in a can promising easy success, but the chances of the contents producing a colorful, carefree meadow are slender.

In first place, the elements are against establishing plants from seed broadcast on newly plowed soil, especially on a slope. Mary's wildflower meadow was twice washed down the hill by heavy rains.

The second challenge meadow makers face is an uphill battle with woody plants. Wherever trees are the climax vegetation, any meadow is a stage in the development of woodland. Seedlings from the native nearby trees invade and take over.

❧ Maintaining a gardener's interpretation of a meadow

This meadow requires considerable maintenance in the form of removing aggressive native perennials like goldenrod, woody plants like sumac, and nonnatives like the multiflora roses.

However, Mary's meadow is an environmentally friendly way to manage a large area without pesticides, fertilizers, or irrigation. And one mowing a year keeps it manageable.

❧ An easier way to make a meadow

Kim Proctor, who did the drawings for this book, and her husband, David, took a very different approach to meadow making. Their goal was simply to reduce the time David spent cutting grass on weekends.

They selected an area of lawn, scratched up patches to expose the soil, ordered seed from Ernst Conservation Seeds, and sowed it in the bare patches. Otherwise, they did nothing except refrain from mowing that part of the lawn.

By midsummer, cosmos and coreopsis flowers from the mix appeared among the long grasses, along with patches of yarrow that had been there all along but had never before had a chance to mature and flower. Even the different kinds of grass proved to be more interesting than they expected, with varying colors, heights, textures, and seed heads.

❧ Maintaining a simple meadow

Twice during the summer, Kim and David forged
through the long grass to remove large weeds. Eventually,
woody plants and aggressive native perennials could be a
problem, but not yet.

At the end of the season, David raised the mower deck
to its highest setting and cut the meadow. Mowing with
the lawn mower wasn't easy, and this year he is thinking
about renting a brush cutter for the day. Otherwise, the
meadow has been as carefree as they had hoped.

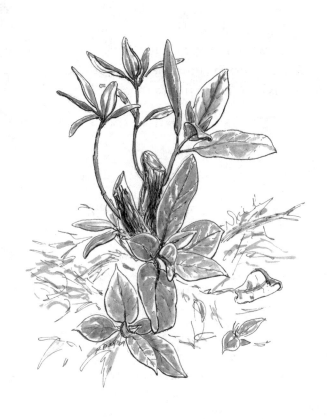

10

Pick Your Battles:
Managing Mature Plants

"THE SUM OF the activities of plants and animals" is one definition of *life* given in *The Chambers Dictionary*. Activities imply motion. And according to Sir Isaac Newton's third law of motion, to every action there is an equal and opposite reaction. Thus, gardeners, acting and reacting, are propelled ever forward, which explains why a garden is never finished. It's always in motion.

As young gardeners, we put in youthful plants that proceed to grow in unexpected and often unintended ways. Suddenly, or so it seems, we become older gardeners and find ourselves trying to control the unwanted but perfectly natural behavior of mature plants. In response, we either accept or resist the changes that have taken place.

If we knew enough or were lucky enough to have put the right plant in the right place, we might not be called upon to do anything for many years. But most of us make mistakes early on and are obliged to cope with the consequences later, which means hanging on to some plants and letting go of others. That's how nature balances the activities of plants and animals—by constantly giving here and taking there.

In the garden, I used to fight against giving an inch and tried to hang on to everything, from ailing plants to crisply cut edges around all the beds. But in the last few years, I have lost many beloved plants to old age and had to relax my death grip on a standard of maintenance well beyond my resources. However, my willingness to accept nature's giving and taking has limits.

The juniper hedge is a case in point. It was planted in 1963 to stabilize and cover up a bank of fill. The young Pfitzer junipers (*Juniperus* ×*pfitzeriana*) took hold immediately. Being sun lovers, they were a suitable choice for the bank, which is exposed to the sun all day. They also proved drought resistant and, fortunately, tolerant of heavy pruning.

As time went by, the junipers wove themselves into a massive informal hedge, which even with regular pruning is hard to maintain at five feet high and fifteen to twenty feet wide. The junipers just keep on growing. And we keep on cutting them back—again and again and again.

Where the hedge meets the upper lawn, its feathery growth habit has been coerced into a soft but straight line that forms the axis of the garden. I can't let that go. But where the ground-sweeping branches reach down the hill to the lower lawn, the edge can be left loose and wavy. These days, pruning the juniper hedge takes far too much time and energy for Erica and me, and having the work done professionally is expensive because it requires skill. But I will hang on to this hedge as long as possible and let go of something else.

At about the same time we planted the junipers, we put in a row of hemlocks along the access road to the state forest. We wanted the privacy that evergreens afford and liked hemlocks for their fine texture. As they are common native trees in the Northeast and grow wild in the state forest, we were sure they would do well.

We planted the young trees about four feet apart in a row, sunny at one end, overhung by a maple tree at the other. I wasn't worried about the shady end because hemlocks had to be shade tolerant; otherwise they wouldn't be at home in the woods. What I didn't know about them was that they can take shade but not dry conditions. And the maple, with its vast root system, was soaking up every drop of moisture in the soil.

I did notice that the hemlocks nearest the maple were growing more slowly than those at the opposite end of the hedge. But by that time, there was such a lot more garden to occupy my thoughts that I'm afraid I rather forgot about the poor hemlocks. So as a result of neglect, the whole hedge eventually grew unkempt, unruly, and finally unmanageable. When I did get someone to prune it from a tall ladder, it took many hours—too many. And recently, wooly adelgid has been added to the hemlock's woes. I am now awaiting the verdict of a professional arborist.

The question is whether the healthiest of the hemlocks are worth saving and at what price. I already know that two or three of the weaker ones will have to go, which raises another issue. Not only have the hemlocks been furnishing a degree of privacy for all these years, they have also been hiding the wire fence that keeps deer out and dogs in. What will I do without this visual barrier? At the moment I don't know, but the arborist may shed some light on the situation.

The worst-case scenario would be to lose all the trees and have to replace them with a wooden fence. Expensive and initially raw looking, a wooden fence might not be too bad if it weathered to a neutral gray. I could always plant in front of it. And one advantage of a solid wooden fence is low maintenance, unless of course a tree limb falls on it, which does happen. This spring, a huge maple limb crashed down on the tall picket fence by the barn and shattered two sections and half of the gate.

But back to the hemlock hedge. The hemlocks present the kind of dilemma that is common in old gardens. The options are not appealing and ardent gardeners resist letting go, but there are times when you might as well bite the bullet. I don't know yet if this is one of them.

In the case of overgrown rhododendrons, I do know from experience that they can actually be rejuvenated by the most savage pruning. It seems like a miracle, but if you cut even huge old giants right to the ground at the end of April or early in May, the stubs will soon leaf out. Within three or four years, you will have lower but denser and more attractive-looking shrubs. I've done it more than once.

You can easily keep these smaller shrubs neat and shapely by pinching off the new terminal growth buds that appear at the ends of the branches. Nip them off while they are still soft, pale green, and only a couple of inches long. This will encourage the plants to put out several side buds and result in bushier, more compact shrubs. Old azaleas, which belong to the genus *Rhododendron*, and closely related mountain laurels, members of the genus *Kalmia*, also respond favorably to this kind of extreme spring pruning.

Of the needled evergreens, only old yews can be revitalized by such harsh means. Otherwise, the rule of thumb with most needled evergreens is to reduce their size by no more than a third in a single season. With very old foundation plantings, you might even consider letting them go rather than hacking away at them every year. It's usually a waste of time and energy.

The hardest decision with shrubs comes not when they are ancient and ugly but when they are approaching maturity and are, for the moment, in perfect harmony and scale with the garden. To keep them this way in the future will require regular pruning, which is time-consuming and ultimately hard on the hands. The alternative is to allow them to keep growing and see what happens. Some will surprise you by remaining shapely, others will not.

To prune or not to prune—that is the question confronting my friend, Rita Buchanan. She is one of the most knowledgeable and talented gardeners I know and has grown most of her trees and shrubs from seed or else from "pups" so tiny that they have had to be coaxed along in a nursery bed. It's no wonder she takes a mother's pride in her woody plants and loves to prune.

During the growing season, Rita spends every waking moment tending the large, beautiful fifteen-year-old garden that she has created with her husband, Steve, but she has another consuming passion. She is a gifted fiber artist and weaver. During the long northwestern Connecticut winters, she works in her studio, producing elegant textiles and utilitarian objects of great beauty.

Looking outside, the gardener in Rita says that she must keep after her shrubs and trees to maintain their ideal proportions. But an artist has only one pair of hands, on which pruning and the hours of repetitive motion take a toll. I don't know what she will decide to do. And probably she doesn't either. Even Rita, with an advanced degree in botany and a lifetime of gardening experience, doesn't have all the answers. But she understands the questions and enjoys the challenge of grappling with them. In the end, we all have to find our own answers. What works for Rita in her garden or me in mine won't necessarily work for you in yours.

In the push-me pull-you world of the aging garden and the aging gardener, the hardest choices involve large trees. Sometimes nature takes a hand in the decision, and an old specimen falls victim to an ice storm or hurricane. If the damage is beyond repair, you will know what to do. But if there is any hope, you will have to decide whether to hang on or let go, considering the age and general health of the tree and its size.

If it's a big tree, you will need the services of a licensed arborist no matter what you decide, and it will be expensive. Expert tree work costs money because it requires knowledge, training, skill, and heavy equipment. And it is dangerous. It's one thing to cut up a fallen tree and something quite else to work off the ground. Two strong young men, experienced with chain saws, cut up the huge maple limb that fell on my picket fence, but down the road I'm facing the loss of the whole tree, which overhangs the barn. Then I will need the Connecticut Arborists, Inc.

Last summer, nature administered the coup de grâce to one of my favorite trees, an old Japanese fantail willow, *Salix udensis* 'Sekka', planted in 1970. While 'Sekka' could also be considered a very large shrub, it had a treelike presence in the garden and a wonderful, almost prehistoric quality. From the base several mighty trunks grew upward and outward, becoming more and more gnarled and twisted with curious, warty protuberances all along the heavy branches. Visitors were always fascinated by the bumps and mystified by the tree's identity. Had they noticed the flattened, curled tips of the branches, they might have recognized it as the willow that flower arrangers use in their designs.

I wasn't alone in my sadness over losing 'Sekka'. Everyone who comes to the garden mourns that plant. At first, I had to steel myself to look at the huge hole it left in the landscape. Then an odd thing happened. I began to get used to the new view of the barn, the crescent bed, and the cluster of winterberry that had been hidden for so many years. I even began to like it. While I would never willingly have parted with the Japanese fantail

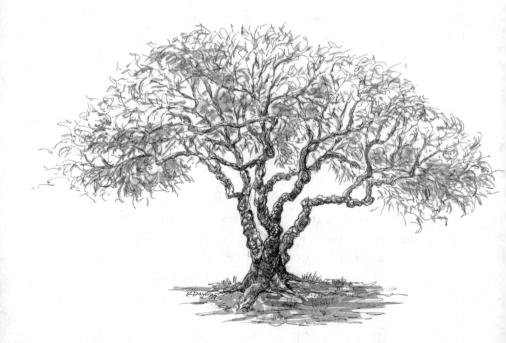

willow, I have come around to the new look. In fact, the spaciousness of the lower lawn now seems like a sigh of relief, a breather from the complexity of beds and borders.

Only a year before the Japanese fantail willow went to its reward, I made the really difficult decision to cut down another favorite tree, a thirty-year-old weeping Higan cherry (*Prunus sub-hirtella* 'Pendula'). Given to me by a great friend in memory of my mother, it was ravishingly beautiful as a young thing, a bower of pale pink blossoms in May and in the fall a cascade of golden-orange leaves. Even in the winter, its graceful lines made a contribution to the garden. But time was not kind to the cherry.

In his definitive *Manual of Woody Landscape Plants*, Michael Dirr says that the Higan cherry is one of the hardier and longer lived of the cherries but that as a breed they are prone to disease and insect damage. I suspect borers in the case of my tree. There were wounds in the bark that had been oozing amber sap for several years. And gradually twigs and branches began to die off and litter the ground. So with a sharp pang of regret, I saw it felled and hauled away.

However, my sorrow at losing the cherry was balanced by my pleasure in seeing the field behind it for the first time in years. I began planting daffodils in the field in 1981 and every spring since have divided a few of the most vigorous and added a few new ones in the fall. But it had been a long time since I had seen them bloom. Suddenly, in the absence of the cherry, I could look out of the windows and see from my office and from the kitchen "a host of golden daffodils."

Another unexpected result of removing the cherry was that the whole of bed A now lay in full view and was flooded with sunlight. Inspired by the possibilities this offered, I imposed yet again upon the kindness of Terence Farrell to help me extend the bed a few feet to accommodate a handsome dwarf blue spruce (*Picea pungens* 'Montgomery').

So life in an old garden isn't all Sturm und Drang. The simplifying process can actually offer opportunities. By not attempting to replace the lost trees, I've gained light and space, which has allowed me to acquire a couple of wonderful new shrubs. But don't feel compelled to replace trees or fill in every hole that appears in your landscape. You may find that you get a better idea or actually prefer the open space.

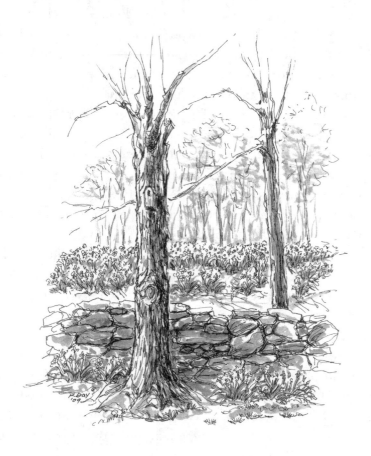

❧ GLEANINGS ❧

❧ Responding to change

Action and reaction is the law of forward motion, and gardens are always moving on. Gardeners plant; plants react by growing; gardeners, in turn, respond either by letting the plants continue to grow or by trying to control their growth.

These actions and reactions have been in progress for so long in my garden that some plants are beyond my ability to manage. A choice must be made to either hang on, which can be a costly battle, or let go, which can be sad.

❧ Choosing your battles

One battleground has been the forty-six-year-old juniper hedge that forms the axis of the whole garden. I feel that fighting to keep the hedge pruned is worth the price.

The fate of a hemlock hedge still hangs in the balance, but I'm leaning toward preservation. Wooly adelgid proves to be not too difficult or expensive to control with oil spray, so I'll give the hedge a chance.

With badly overgrown rhododendrons, azaleas, and mountain laurels, the choice is easy: let go and the sooner the better. Brutal pruning, right to the ground, done early in the spring can renew and revitalize the plants.

Of the needled evergreens, only yews recover from such drastic pruning. The rest take more kindly to being reduced in size gradually and over a period of years.

❧ Controlling plant growth by pruning

Reducing or maintaining a certain size and dimensions by pruning requires attention to the line, branching pattern, structure, shape, and form of each plant. Try not to violate the plant's natural shape.

Working with loppers and pruners is satisfying, but unfortunately the repetitive motion involved is hard on your hands. Older gardeners beware. You've only got one pair of hands. So, again, choose your subjects for pruning carefully. Not all shrubs demand it.

You might try limiting the number of specimens that *have* to be pruned and letting the rest do their own thing. The trick is to prune enough to keep plants in scale but not enough to ruin your hands.

❧ Hard choices

It's hard to bear the loss of old trees that have made a positive contribution to the garden for many years. But sometimes their removal is necessary to preserve buildings and protect other plantings from damage. Declining health is another reason to remove full-grown trees, and it can be a difficult choice that has to be weighed. A lot depends on the age and health of the tree.

In the aftermath of losing a big tree, don't be in too great a hurry to replace it or fill the gap in your landscape. You may find that you like the open space.

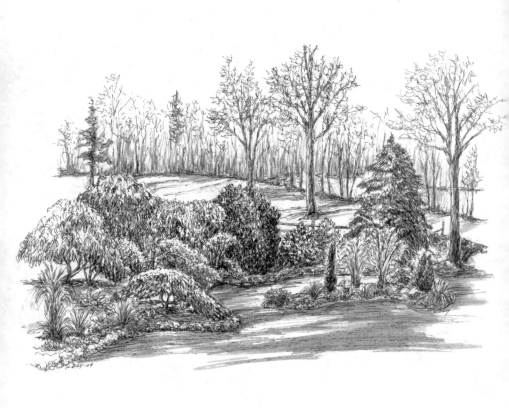

11

What Next?
Deciding Whether to Stay Put or Move On

ON THE LAST Sunday in March 2009, I walked every inch of the property. At this time of year, my favorite place is the woodland garden, where the aconites had almost finished their cheerful flowering. Already, a few red-purple blossoms of *Primula abschasica* from Linc and Timmy Foster hovered above the dead leaves. Soon there would be many more. This species from the Caucasus has always been the first to flower and the most enduring of all the primroses, tolerant of winter cold, summer heat, and even drought.

Along the stream, the shiny black-green foliage of marsh marigolds had formed low mounds. The round buds and gleaming yellow flowers were still a couple of weeks away. But a dry winter had already reduced the stream to a trickle. It makes me nervous when the water table is as low as this so early in the season.

The woodland garden was my next-to-last stop on this slow meander through the garden, slow partly because a hip complaint had hobbled me for the last ten days. Nevertheless, I managed to go either up or down all the steps, most of which are homemade and some in need of shoring up. My route took me past the old stile in the stone wall. Flat slabs of fieldstone project just enough to serve as steps and provide access to the field above.

I uncovered the stile more than forty years ago while stripping the wall of woodbine and poison ivy. Later, when we were driven to put up the deer fence, we made a gate in the wire netting so that the stile would still be accessible. But time passed and the rhododendrons grew, obscuring and finally hiding the stile completely. However, it occurred to me on that Sunday that it would be quite easy to open up a tunnel under these huge shrubs by taking out a few branches. It was a tempting thought.

The path among the rhododendrons brought me down onto the lawn at the far end of the garden, where I passed behind beds A and B on my way to the woodland garden. Leaving the woods, I continued south past the crescent bed. The transition to shrub border was almost complete, and I was pleased to see that the new *Chamaecyparis obtusa* 'Nana Gracilis' had come through the winter with flying colors. Continuing around the perimeter of the lower lawn, I stopped to inspect the handiwork of the Connecticut Arborists, Inc.

I had come to a decision about the hemlocks. After learning that controlling the wooly adelgid was not prohibitively expensive, I voted in favor of salvaging as much of the hedge as possible. As I was stuck with the hemlocks, the first step was to begin cutting them back, an ongoing process that will take two or three years. Stage 1 has now been completed, and the hedge is four feet shorter. Later two men will return and take out the worst-looking and unhappiest of the hemlocks. A few are beyond hope.

While I had an arborist in the garden, I seized the moment and had the juniper hedge trimmed, just the edge along the upper lawn, which is now clean and straight and looks a thousand times better. Getting the two big hedges into some kind of order raised my spirits, which had taken a hit when I realized how inhibiting my hip was going to be. At the moment, I'm useless in the garden.

While the pruning was not cheap, the price was reasonable for expert work. But any additional pruning this year will depend on the state of my body and on how successful Erica and I have been in making the rest of the garden less demanding. Terence, our secret weapon, has already been invaluable in the pruning department. He recently worked wonders with the *Heptacodium miconioides*. It can become a shaggy, rather unkempt tree that eventually reaches twenty feet or more. Over the years I've coaxed this one into a relatively low umbrella shape, which Terence has refined. The sweetly scented August-blooming flowers give this tree its odd common name of seven-son flower. The clusters of small white blossoms, borne in six-flowered tiers, terminate in a single slightly larger blossom, presumably the seventh son. The sepals remain long after the flowers are gone and turn a lovely cherry red. These and the late season of bloom make a real contribution to the shrub border.

Besides assessing my progress in simplifying the garden, the weekend walkabout had a larger purpose. I wanted to look at the big picture with as objective an eye as possible in order to understand what I must do next in order to stay here.

Two friends of mine, whom you will meet shortly, have re-

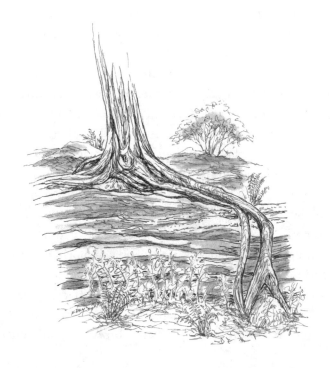

cently moved and left behind very large and much loved gardens. Both are happy with their decisions, one deliriously so and the other quietly confident that it was the right thing to do. Both love the new gardens they are making. I wish I could be as sure about what I'm doing. But simplification is a work in progress, and I'm acutely aware that I don't know how it will turn out.

When I was in my teens, I embarked on writing the Great American Novel. It would, of course, have been a thinly disguised family portrait, and the beginning chapters—about my brothers, my parents, and our numerous pets—were easy. But time and again, I foundered when I realized that I didn't know how the story ended. Nor could I stretch my imagination enough to invent an ending. I wasn't a fiction writer at heart.

Today I'm in a similar predicament, because in telling the real story of this garden, I don't know the ending. Gardens don't have endings like novels. And as gardeners, we don't want them to be finished. In any case, real life works in ways we cannot anticipate and will never understand. It continues to evolve, leaving gaps, holes, and loose ends as it unfolds. But I do know one thing—I'm not moving if I can help it.

My past is woven too deeply into this familiar landscape, which reminds me so much of home. This was my world growing up. Our neighbors were farmers who scraped a living out of skimpy soil that barely covers the bedrock. Their lives were dominated by work, weather, and the changing seasons. Early exposure to this kind of life must have rubbed off on me, because I've chosen a version of it myself. Although an Englishman is never anything but an Englishman, Martin also chose to live in Connecticut and to put down roots here. Like those of a couple of old trees, our roots became intertwined, anchoring us to each other and to this place. This is where we belong.

On the four and a half acres of woodland across from the house, there are several high ridges where exposed bedrock has cracked and tree seedlings have taken root. Against all odds, the seedlings have grown into trees, forcing apart slabs of the bedrock, which break away and give the ridges their angular silhouettes. From a flat spot in the middle of one of the ridges, there are fine views in every direction: to the north higher and higher rocky ledges, and to the east the garden spread out below and glimpses of Lake Lillinonah through the bare trees.

Ethan Currier, a talented young stone sculptor, created the beautiful granite bench that now takes advantage of the views. Five powerful men hauled and rolled the bench end over end through the woods, up the steep incline, and into its place. As it came to rest, one of the five took out a level and laid it along the top. It was absolutely perfect. Martin's name is carved into the stone. That's another reason I don't anticipate leaving here. But when I do, the land will be protected from development because it has been deeded to the Newtown Forest Association.

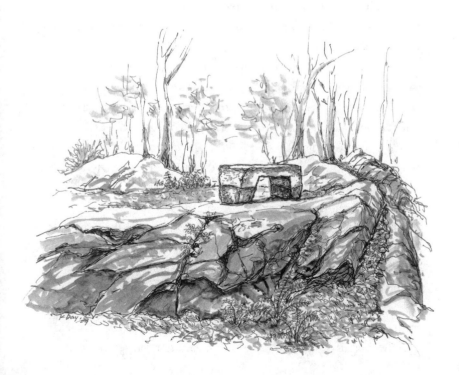

So far, staying put has seemed the right decision for me, but it would not have been right for my young friend and neighbor Martha McKeon. Five years after her husband's death in 1999, Martha pulled up stakes and quit the huge garden she had been trying to manage by herself. It was sad for Martin and me because we were very attached to Martha and her family, and the garden she left behind was lovely. She and Bill had been working on it for years.

Our introduction to the McKeons was a charming note from Martha saying that she had enjoyed my first book, *A Patchwork Garden*. "I would love to see your garden," she wrote, "and also have you come to our place, where we have attempted to make some sense of our Connecticut wilderness."

By the following year when I finally got over to see the garden, she and Bill had done a great deal more than tame their four acres of wilderness, which included a brook and a pond. They had developed an attractive perennial bed around a flowering dogwood, had planted a small rose garden, and were working on an ambitious border that would eventually run all the way down one side of the property from the house to the pond.

Martin and I were very taken with the McKeons, their garden, and their offspring. Our refrigerator was soon festooned with Libby's and Sarah's artwork and an award bestowed on Martin for "telling the best jokes." It was a treat to find such lively, kind, amusing young friends in our own backyard! Bill was always performing services for us, and Martha often came and helped me in the garden.

Tragedy struck in 1999 with Bill's sudden death, which devastated the family and their many friends. Although Martha carried on with indomitable strength and spirit, her life was very much changed and the property soon became a burden. "It just got to be too much," she says now, "and I had no time for anything else."

She began looking for a much smaller place in Stratford,

Connecticut, where her friend and business partner, Anne Lees, lives with her husband, Steve. The two women design and install landscapes and maintain them for their clients. Martha had been going to visit Anne and Steve for years and always liked the town. She describes Stratford as "a cozy place, where people live in the same houses for fifty years."

Fortunately, she was able to sell her Newtown property before the real estate market collapsed. And when she realized that she could now afford a small house in a lovely section called Lordship, within blocks of Long Island Sound, it all came together. At the end of a mile-and-a-half-long causeway, across acres of marsh grass and saltwater inlets, Lordship has been overlooked by time and change. All the houses are small, neat, and simple. Most are well kept with handkerchief-sized front lawns and usually a tree or two.

Martha's requirements were a Cape Cod–style house on a fifty-by-one-hundred-foot lot—no bigger. "Most people are looking for space and privacy," she says, "but I was looking for the opposite. I was tired of being so isolated, and I had made the garden too big." Now she has the best of both worlds, a friendly neighborhood and a beautiful, manageable garden entirely enclosed by a weathered Nantucket picket fence. "I like it a lot here," she says, "and so do the kids. Libby is still living with me, and Sarah is about two minutes away." Cole, Sarah's little son, is a recent addition and frequent visitor with his mother. So once again, life is good for Martha and the family.

Mary Ann McGourty's move from the nursery that she and her husband started in 1978 and ran for twenty-two years was shorter in distance but no less wrenching than Martha's. Fred, Mary Ann's husband and partner of thirty years, died the year after Martin.

I had known the McGourtys since 1980 and admired them both. At that time, I was taking classes from Fred at the New York Botanical Garden, where he became the first recipient of the Distinguished Educator in Plant Studies award. Everybody loved Fred's classes. He had the ability to convey information clearly, concisely, and always amusingly. You never forgot the plants that he dubbed "thugs" or failed to understand the implications of growing perennials, which he defined as "plants that come up every year, if they live." In other words, not all perennials are reliably perennial.

For all his years of experience and training—he held degrees from the University of Pennsylvania and New York University—and the honors heaped upon him, Fred remained the same. He never forgot that he was first and foremost a home gardener, and he made other home gardeners his priority. He educated us, introduced us to new and interesting plants through the nursery, and made us better gardeners by example and by his teaching and writing.

Fred's death in 2006 was a loss to the entire gardening world. His former college roommate and lifelong friend called him "a national treasure." But he couldn't have done what he did without Mary Ann. They were partners in the nursery business; they both designed gardens for clients; and they shared a close, affectionate domesticity that warmed the hearts of everyone who knew them. Physically mismatched—Mary Ann tall and thin; Fred much shorter, distinctly round and cherubic—they fit together perfectly as companions, highly intelligent, warm, kind, funny, and unpretentious.

Even before they closed the nursery in 2000, Mary Ann knew that living at Hillside would eventually become too much for them. The garden, which had also been the display and demonstration garden for the nursery, covered five acres and consisted of twenty perennial borders. "It simply wasn't possible to keep it up," she said recently. "While we still had the nursery, we were able to write off garden help as a business expense, but now we couldn't afford that kind of help."

By this time, Fred's health had begun to deteriorate, and she started gently nudging him toward a smaller place and a less stressful life. Eventually he came around and gave her the go-ahead to start looking for a smaller house and a few acres in nearby Norfolk, Connecticut. Although he never lived there, he liked the house she found and put his stamp of approval on it.

Simple, well built, and attractive, Mary Ann's new home sits comfortably on a wooded knoll with an apron of lawn around it, and beyond the lawn the beautiful northwestern Connecticut woodland landscape drops away to the east and south. Of the three acres, two and a half will remain wooded. But around the house, a few old Norway spruces have been felled, and a new garden is already well under way. Fred would be pleased.

❧ GLEANINGS ❧

❧ Assessing progress

In the spring of 2009, I needed to assess the progress Erica and I had made the summer before in making the garden easier to maintain. Walking around the property and checking up on works in progress made me hopeful about the future. There's no telling whether my early decision to stay put will prove to be the right one, but so far it feels right.

Before Martin's death, I felt that I would want to stay here and live in the house we found together and in which we invested ourselves. The house is surrounded by a landscape that he loved and over the years helped make. The garden has brought me friends, a modest form of artistic expression, and an even more modest source of income. The bottom line is that I am happy here and seem to be managing, after a fashion.

❧ The major decision

Losing a beloved spouse shatters your life. Martha McKeon and Mary Ann McGourty have been through it, Mary Ann most recently. What to do next is a hard decision, and you have to make it on your own.

Sympathetic people will tell you that they know how you feel. But you are the only one who really knows and can figure out what to do. No one can advise you—not your children, not your friends, not your financial advisor or attorney.

You just have to hang on, listen to your heart, and trust your gut. That's what Martha, Mary Ann, and I have all done, each in our own way.

❧ Martha's decision

By the time Martha had spent five years commuting an hour and a half to work every day, bringing up two teenage daughters on her own, and trying to keep up the large garden that she and Bill had maintained together, she'd had enough.

While Bill was alive, Newtown was a good place to live, but as a single woman she found their place too isolated and herself too busy to have a life. What she wanted was a small house on a small lot in a town near her work.

With the stars propitiously aligned, she sold her Newtown property and found a new home in Stratford, Connecticut, near her friend and business partner, Anne. The new house and garden fit her to a T.

❧ Mary Ann's decision

Mary Ann had seen the writing on the wall as early as 2000, the year she and Fred closed Hillside Gardens, the nursery they had established and managed together for twenty-two years. Their garden had also been the nursery display garden, and without the nursery staff, five acres and twenty perennial borders could not be maintained.

By this time Fred's health had deteriorated, and Mary Ann felt that a smaller place and less work would be better for them both. Although he never lived in the house she found in nearby Norfolk, Connecticut, he saw it and put his stamp of approval on it. She knew that it was the right thing to do. And now she is in the process of making a new garden, reasonable in size and close to the house.

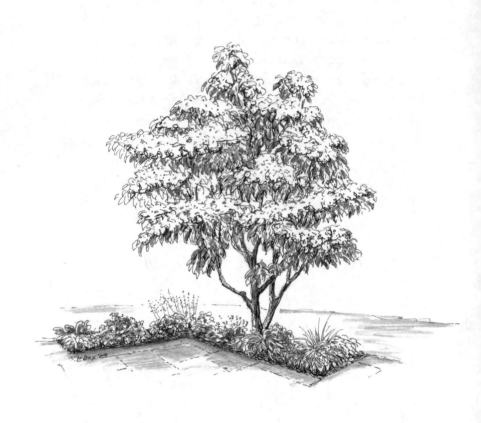

12

New Gardens:
Keeping Them Small and Simple

NOT LONG AFTER taking stock of my own situation, I visited Mary Ann McGourty at her new home. While southern Connecticut had been luxuriating in a few springlike days, here in the northwest corner of the state substantial piles of snow lingered in the shade. Norfolk claims the title "The Icebox of Connecticut" and proudly flaunts it on little blue and white banners that fly from every lamppost along Main Street.

Mountainous and still rural, Norfolk is in one of the loveliest parts of this very pretty old state, and Mary Ann has found herself a perfect spot about a mile and a half from town. The house enjoys complete privacy, concealed from the road by a wooded hillside and from the only visible house to the north by a felicitous grouping of hemlocks and shrubs. Mary Ann met me in the driveway and pointed to the foot of the slope, where she had already begun planting.

"The first thing I did when I came here," she said, "was to take out five huge old Norway spruces. They were covering the whole hillside and looming over the house. Besides the spruces, there were shrubs in front of every window. So after the trees went, I dug up all the shrubs and replanted them halfway up the hill. Then I put in these new low-growing spireas, a short white fothergilla, and in front of them a couple of little weigelas. The idea is that the new shrubs will spread out and cover the lower slope. Eventually the perennial ground covers, like *Phlox subulata* and that wonderful *Veronica* 'Aztec Gold', will completely fill in among them."

This slope, which faces the front of the house, already looked well established to me, but Mary Ann described it as a work in progress. She has plans to remove the rooted layers from a large rhododendron, which is taking up valuable space. "Then," she says, "I'll have a place for some more new things, mostly low shrubs, glued together with whatever ground covers seem appropriate."

One of the things that appealed to me was the way the rest of the beds hugged the house. Under the kitchen windows, two heavily fruiting winterberries with some of their red berries still intact shared space with their male pollinator, and in front of them were planted peonies and Siberian irises for early summer color.

Moving around the house from bed to bed, Mary Ann pointed out plants that she had saved from the previous owner's garden. "I thought I ought to have a little something from Mrs. Dockham's garden, like this Korean spice viburnum. It's rather

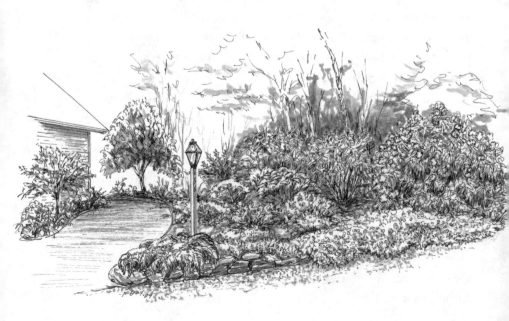

ordinary most of the year, but you love it to death when it's in bloom because of the wonderful fragrance."

Arriving at a sheltered flagstone terrace, I recognized familiar faces from Hillside Gardens, Mary Ann's former home. During the eighties and nineties, gardeners from all over New England made regular pilgrimages to the McGourty's nursery to admire and to learn. The display gardens around their eighteenth-century farmhouse offered valuable lessons in how to use the plants available at the nursery. Just wandering around among the beds was an education, but the best part of a visit was that one of the McGourtys was usually on hand to offer advice or guidance.

It was reassuring to see masses of *Geranium macrorrhizum* from Hillside along Mary Ann's new driveway, and around the house other McGourty favorites including their selection of *Aruncus aethusifolius, Carex elata* 'Bowles Golden' (a low, grassy sedge with golden-striped leaves), *Epimedium* 'Bandit', variegated brunnera, Japanese painted fern, and European ginger. At one corner of the terrace a handsome *Cornus kousa* protects these shade dwellers from the southern sun.

By lunchtime we had explored the garden and were ready to come indoors, where the pale March sunshine poured through unobstructed windows. With the shrubs gone and the overhanging spruces a thing of the past, the rooms are filled with light. After lunch we were joined in the living room by the two Maine coon cats with whom Mary Ann shares her house and life, and she reminisced about starting the nursery.

Harold Epstein, a towering figure in the North American Rock Garden Society who collected plants from all over the world, had been instrumental in pointing the McGourtys in the right direction. "When Harold gave us starts of about a dozen of his best plants, we recognized our niche immediately," said Mary Ann. "What was going to make our nursery different from other nurseries was offering unique or little-known plants. People were not going to come here to buy daisies, but they would come for

unusual woodlanders like *Deinanthe bifida*, a herbaceous relative of hydrangea, or some of the sedges and grasses, which were
very new at that time."

Later we discussed some of the challenges of older gardens
and older gardeners, because whether you decide to stick with
the devil known or move to a smaller property, you still have
major decisions to make. At some point in the conversation, I
discovered that she does a talk called "Downsizing a Large Garden" in which she describes the approach she has taken.

"Two things were instrumental in keeping this garden more
manageable," she says. "The first was making the decision to
stick primarily to bulbs, which virtually take care of themselves,
and to use a lot of ground covers and shrubs. The big difference
is that at Hillside, we had five acres of perennials, and at first I
thought I had to bring all Fred's and my favorites with me. But
there were so many. The problem then became, which of them
should I bring?

"So the second thing I decided was to choose a color scheme,
and that has helped me make some kind of order out of all this.
I had designed so many pastel gardens for other people that my
first thought was no more pink, mauve, and lavender. This garden is mostly blue, yellow, and white. That palette has helped me
a lot in narrowing down what to bring. Of course, a few other
colors have crept in. The *Spiraea japonica* 'Alpina' was already in
before I figured out that I wasn't going to have any pink."

I couldn't agree with Mary Ann more about the benefits of a
limited palette. By confining your color scheme to a few com-
patible hues, you will greatly simplify your life and your garden.
The effect of the garden itself will be more cohesive, and the
temptations fewer. I learned this from making container gardens
with a set color scheme.

Another important decision Mary Ann made was to strictly
limit the number of perennials in her new garden. Aside from
the perennial ground covers used in the hillside planting and the

few favorites around the terrace, Mary Ann has stuck to her plan. However, she made one exception. At the top of the driveway lies a long, narrow strip of garden filled with daylilies. Mary Ann is a lady after my own heart! I couldn't garden without daylilies. Hers are underplanted with daffodil bulbs, a symbiotic pairing that provides two seasons of bloom and solves the problem of the spent daffodil foliage. The arching leaves of the daylilies soon cover it up completely.

Mary Ann is thinking about planting more daffodils in the surrounding woods and may add wildflowers to the existing native plants. Her treasured double bloodroot and double trillium from Hillside have already made themselves at home in the wooded area at the foot of her driveway.

When I told Mary Ann how much I liked everything she had done, she smiled and said, "Well, this has been my therapy. It's gotten me through two and a half years. And there is plenty more to do. I've had fun thinking about it and planning it, and there has been the comfort of having the things Fred and I loved at Hillside. But there are also the new things that are me, establishing myself here."

Then Mary Ann laughed and added, "I've only done a few things that I think would make Fred really roll his eyes. The most visible is the steel edging, but it does help keep grass out of the beds and it keeps me from doing things that I shouldn't do, such as making the beds bigger! The other thing he wouldn't like is the *Buddleja*. Fred was *not* a fan of butterfly bush in this climate. We're on the edge of its hardiness range, but I've got a dwarf variety three feet tall, and it's the only thing, except for the Japanese maple, that I have to cosset.

"Otherwise, getting ready for winter here is easy. I only have a few perennials to cut down, a bit of chicken wire to put round the butterfly bush and stuff with leaves, and the trunk of the Japanese maple to wrap. The guy that mows the lawn just blows the leaves into the woods. So that's the story." It's a story of success, the durability of the human spirit, and the long-lasting pleasures of gardening.

Martha McKeon's story is similar in many ways but also very different. Gardens woven from the threads of a real life, from the heart, soul, and experiences of an individual, are always unique. You get to know gardeners best, and at their best, through their gardens. An invitation to someone's garden is a personal offering, a gift of self. For ten years I had the privilege and pleasure of seeing Martha and her garden often. And I watched her grow and mature as a gardener and as a person. From the start it was obvious that she had what it took—the physical strength and optimism of the typical gardener—and something else that has stood her in good stead, a realistic view of life and gardens and a sense of humor.

Her English grandfather came to America as a young man and became head gardener on the Westchester County, New York, estate where Martha grew up. He won prizes galore at flower shows and became best known for his roses. But he never lost his down-to-earth approach to horticulture: hard work produced good plants and good gardens. So Martha had a head start before she even put spade to ground. By the time we knew the McKeons, the stage was set for the increasingly interesting garden the young couple was developing on their wet, wooded site.

Martha's new shoreline property is as different from the four woodland acres she left behind as two places could possibly be. But among the perennials in her new garden, I instantly recognized the daylilies and a few other old standbys I'd grown for years. In her old garden, the main border was roughly translated from English models, Americanized to fit her wet woodland setting and zone 6 conditions. Now these same perennials found themselves tucked and grouped among shrubs and small ornamental trees against a weathered gray picket fence under the wide, uncluttered shoreline sky. Large trees are few and far between so near the coast, and the sky seems bigger. Even on an overcast day the reflected light from the water three blocks away creates a luminous atmosphere.

Rectilinear beds laid out in a formal pattern along the fence and against the wall of the garage bask in the sun. The center of the garden is subdivided into a square vegetable plot with a bird-bath centerpiece. In front of the vegetable garden, three hydrangeas cluster around a dramatically tall clump of Joe Pye weed from Martha's old garden to create the focal point.

In time, the rounded shrubs and fountain of Joe Pye weed will play second fiddle to a magnificent weeping white spruce (*Picea glauca* 'Pendula'), at the moment about ten feet high. A few feet in front of the spruce, a sculpture of iron rings welded into a cantilevered tower mimics the tall, narrow shape of the tree. The rings were one of Bill's dump finds. The garden ends at a small bluestone patio, where Martha has planted a shapely

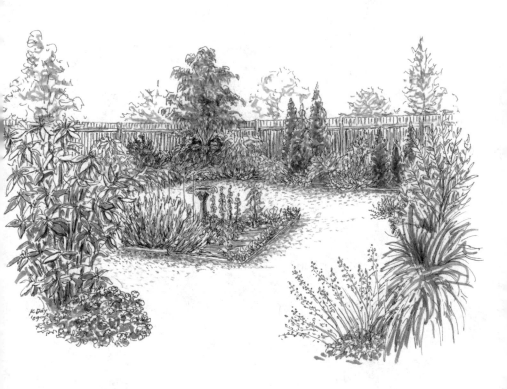

hawthorn tree. Already it is producing enough shade to make the patio cool and pleasant in the summer.

With the misery of the move and the grunt work of potting and transporting her perennials from the old garden fading fast, what remains are the funny stories of Martha's arrival. She describes the horror of her new neighbors when they stopped by to commiserate with her about the dead lawn, only to learn that she had purposely sprayed it with herbicide. Now, in place of struggling lawn with two matching Norway maples growing out of it, the trees stand in neat, no-maintenance squares of ivy on either side of a welcoming front walk.

The entire backyard was subjected to the same treatment and the grass replaced by a grid of garden beds and broad paths of

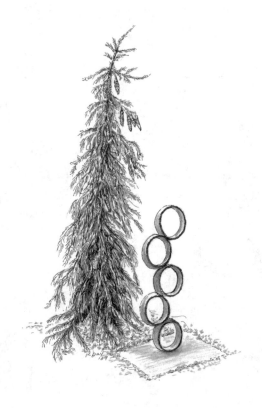

pea gravel. Martha doesn't own such a thing as a mower. When I asked what else had been in the backyard, she grinned. "About five different kinds of fencing in various stages of disrepair, that poor little Japanese maple planted a foot too deep, and a fire hydrant! A *real* fire hydrant!"

The real but nonfunctioning fire hydrant was the first thing to go; the little Japanese maple, one of the lacy red-leaved Dissectum Group, was rescued and properly replanted; and the fence was put in. Martha described the fence color as "that brand-new-wood look," but it only took a year to weather to a lovely soft gray.

That fall she broke her arm and couldn't do anything with the garden, but daughters Libby and Sarah pitched in and got all the plants she had brought from Newtown out of their pots and into the ground. In the spring, with her arm healed, Martha laid out the garden. "It went very quickly," she said. "I pretty much did all the things you had taught me about repetition of the perennials, and I used almost all the same plants. There are only about ten or twelve perennials that Anne and I really like anyway."

These days, Martha and Anne have to use bulletproof plants for their clients' gardens. Even well-to-do clients are watching their budgets, so the women fall back on perennials that they know from experience will give good value all season and for many seasons to come.

When push comes to shove, what makes a garden beautiful is healthy, happy, well-chosen plants arranged in pleasing combinations; and with proper care, but no extreme measures, they should go on performing over an extended period of time. "The foliage has to look good from start to finish," says Martha. "That's the criterion we have to go with. The same with the pots. The stuff has to look decent from May to November. Everybody thinks they want tons of flowers, but they really don't. So even in the containers, we always sneak in a lot of foliage plants."

Martha and Anne have been keeping clients happy with their plant choices for the last ten years. Among the following list of their perennial favorites for the long haul, many will now be familiar to you, and most are plants Mary Ann and I have been using for decades: *Sedum* 'Autumn Joy', daylilies, Siberian irises, catmint, lamb's ears, lily turf, and ornamental grasses. "We use some other little grassy things, too, where the conditions are sometimes too wet or too shady or too dry. For damp places we've been using sweet flag (*Acorus*) a lot, and if it's shady, Japanese forest grass; for sun, if we want something grassy in the front but a little bigger, we use fountain grass. That's about it. And we use tons of shrubs and mix them all together.

"For flowering shrubs, we like a lot of different viburnums and hydrangeas, which do exceptionally well here near the coast in zone 7. Anne and I also love the spiraeas 'Little Princess', 'Gold Mound', and 'Anthony Waterer'. We shear them like boxwoods once or twice a year, and they look great. Incidentally, boxwoods

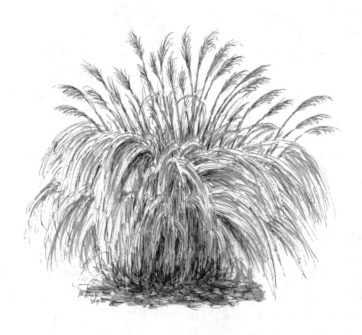

are dynamite down here, too. We don't try to be exotic. We just want things to grow and to be beautiful and to be easy to take care of." That makes four of us: Mary Ann, Martha, Anne, and me, and probably plenty of other people just like us.

✤ GLEANINGS ✤

✤ Starting over

Starting over is not easy, but with years of experience behind them, Mary Ann McGourty and Martha McKeon have succeeded in establishing new gardens in a very short time. Both used plants from their old gardens, which helped. And Mary Ann, who still owned Hillside Gardens at the time she moved, brought along buckets of the rich compost she and Fred had been making for years.

✤ Mary Ann's new, more manageable garden

The first bed Mary Ann showed me was a template for the other beds: a few compact evergreens and dwarf flowering shrubs (like low-growing *Weigela* 'Midnight Wine', cushions of *Spiraea japonica* 'Alpina,' and a short white fothergilla) knitted together by perennial ground covers (like creeping *Phlox subulata* and *Veronica* 'Aztec Gold').

Initially, Mary Ann made two decisions that keep her new garden manageable. The first was to stick to bulbs, which take care of themselves, and to use a lot of shrubs and ground covers. Having left behind five acres of perennial borders, she has exercised caution in adding perennials, though some favorites are now in residence.

While she longed to bring all Fred's and her own favorite perennials, their sheer numbers presented another problem. That's when she decided to choose a color scheme—blue, yellow, and white—and stick to it, which for the most part she has done.

In a lecture she gives on downsizing a large garden, she recommends Jack-in-the-box planting for small spaces—ground covers underplanted with bulbs, and carpets of ground covers at the base of shrubs.

Mary Ann's new garden has gotten her through two and a half difficult years and will continue to be a source of comfort, and not a burden, as she reconstructs her life.

�֍ Martha's new keep-it-simple world

My first glimpse of Martha's new garden was through a throng of people gathered for daughter Sarah's baby shower. It was late September and ornamental grasses waved over the heads of the guests. A picket fence enclosed formal beds, informally planted but with structure and geometry provided by groups of dwarf Alberta spruces and globes of boxwood.

Martha's rule for keeping it simple was to limit the size of the lot, eliminate all lawn, repeat the shrub combination of dwarf Alberta spruces and boxwoods, and use flowering shrubs—especially hydrangeas, viburnums, and spiraeas—to add substance and color. As fillers, she uses a few grasses and perennials from her old garden.

The next time I saw the garden, Sarah's baby was an affable cherub of six months and the perennials were just beginning to emerge from winter dormancy. There were still a few dry stems to cut down, and little troughs of dead leaves edged the gravel paths. Otherwise, the garden looked perfectly tidy. Martha says that spring cleanup now takes her an hour.

❀ **Plant picks from two professional gardeners for easy-care gardens**

The few perennials Martha and her business partner, Anne, use in clients' gardens and their own are easy to grow and have good foliage: *Sedum* 'Autumn Joy', catmint (*Nepeta* ×*faassenii* 'Blue Wonder'), Siberian irises (*Iris sibirica* cultivars), lily turf (*Liriope muscari*), lamb's ears (*Stachys byzantina* 'Silver Carpet'), and ornamental grasses.

Favorite grasses are *Miscanthus udensis* 'Morning Light'; fountain grass (*Pennisetum alopecuroides* 'Hamelin' and 'Little Bunny'); and for shade, Japanese forest grass (*Hakonechloa macra*), a solid green, gently arching grass about a foot tall; and *H. macra* 'Aureola', with a similar habit, only yellow foliage with green stripes.

What Martha and Anne want from their plants is also what Mary Ann and I want. We want them to look attractive and grow without making too many demands.

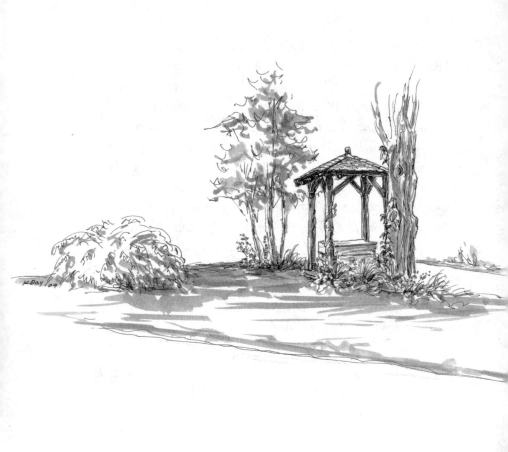

13

Borrowed Landscapes:
Using the Garden Setting

PEOPLE OFTEN ASK how Martin and I found our house. Even now with GPS devices and accurate directions, first-time visitors frequently go astray. If the wanderers are in the immediate neighborhood, someone will point them toward the dirt track up into the state forest, but a few doors down the road no one can help them. The new neighbors come and go too quickly.

My old neighbors all live within a few hundred yards of a grassy triangle where three confusing country roads meet. We have been neighbors and friends for more than forty years. My nearest neighbors are at the bottom of my dirt road. They arrived three years after we did. Another lives a stone's throw away, down the road on the left. And our other neighbors live at the end of a long driveway almost opposite my road. They are the ones most often called upon to send the UPS truck or some other lost soul back up their drive and into the state forest.

When Martin and I came here, cows still grazed in the field across from our nearest neighbor's house. Echo Valley Road is a mile long, and at that time there were only four other houses on it, all built before 1850. Old maps show our house as the last one on the road, which still peters out as it disappears into the woods. The house was built by the Sanford family, and one of the three roads bears their name. Sanford Road has recently been declared a Scenic Road, which means that it will remain unpaved and never be widened or improved. It winds through swampy woodland and comes out on the main road to town. Albert's Hill

Road was also a dirt road in those days, ending at the cove on Lake Lillinonah.

The cove was a gathering place for that generation of teenagers, who built small fires and drank beer there on Saturday nights. No one bothered them. But if they got too loud, the neighbor living nearest to the racket would yell down the hill and the noise would cease—for a while.

Echo Valley Road used to be so far off the beaten track that even Martin, who loved to explore back roads, might never have found it had it not been for our real estate agent, who lived there. We had been house hunting for some time and had found nothing. Then one day in September, Mrs. Knox called to say she had a new listing she wanted to show us but had left the key at home. Would we mind stopping off at her house to pick it up?

Every single thing about the mile we traveled on Echo Valley Road was perfect. We passed a little pond ringed round with swamp maples in their fall regalia and came to the grassy triangle with a rustic well house in the middle of it. From there, we veered off into the woods up the dirt track that looked like a riverbed. And there it was, our dream house, a prim nineteenth-century farmhouse, standing in a circle of sugar maples that were shedding their golden leaves. This was the place we had been looking for.

There was only one snag. The house, its old red barn, and the four acres on which they stood belonged to Isabelle and Bill Knox. And the answer to my first question was, "No, my dear, we have no intention of selling."

Two months went by. We continued to look at houses, but after the fateful day we picked up that key we saw nothing we liked. So it was a stunning surprise when Isabelle Knox called us in November and asked if we were still interested. The reasons she gave for their change of heart were that they were nearing retirement, winter was coming, and she had recently had a bad fall. I also think that our response to the house that they had loved for twenty years influenced their decision, because in the end they even lowered the asking price. On January 26, 1961, we moved in with almost no furniture, a dog, and a large table saw. The rest is the subject of my first book, *A Patchwork Garden*.

Lest you think I'm never going to return to the theme of simpler gardening, there is a point to this rather long story. I have felt drawn to the landscape of Connecticut with almost magnetic force since earliest childhood. Some look to the hills for the sound of the music, but I look to the woods, and in my old age they mean more than ever. That is really why I am telling you all this.

Just beyond the garden walls lies a forest of maple, oak, tulip poplar, sweet birch, and American beech. Groves of hemlock cling to north- and east-facing cliffs above Lake Lillinonah. The Upper Paugussett State Forest covers a bulge of land wrapped round by the Housatonic River, which flows into the lake formed by damming the river about a mile from our house.

In the old days, we used to walk down to watch the eagles

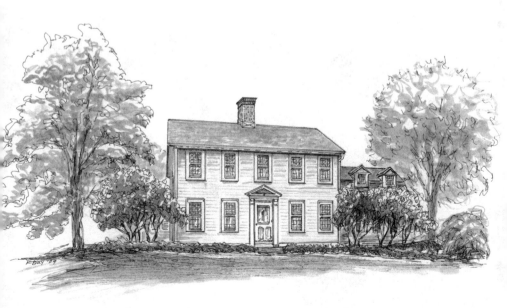

fishing at the bottom of the dam where the water plunged back into the river. Such easy access is no longer permitted. But a generous strip of contiguous woodland follows the downward course of the river, creating a remarkable parcel of open space. In the winter, glimpses of the dam are visible through the trees from the upstairs windows. And from every window, woodland stretches as far as the eye can see. I feel that all of this is mine. What the eye can see, the heart can possess.

I love the trees, individually and collectively. The tulip poplars are as straight as the masts of sailing ships, and the flowers are exquisite but too far up in the canopy to make any kind of show. It is only when they fall to the ground that you can study them closely—the lovely color scheme of cream, yellow, orange, and the freshest of fresh green. Their beautifully fashioned cups of six overlapping petals with a boss of stamens in the middle remind me of anemones.

Most of the oaks have not yet reached an age when they are

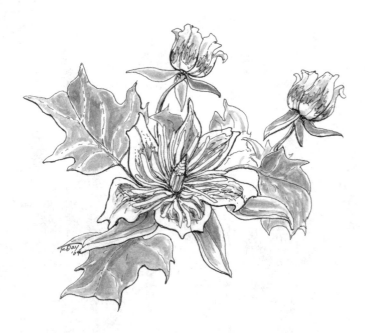

at their most magnificent. After all, this woodland is less than a hundred years old. But sometimes huge, solitary oaks can be found in the middle of the forest, surrounded by younger trees. Majestic survivors from the nineteenth century, these "wolf trees," so called because they usually stand by themselves, took root next to a stone wall or large rock outcrop and thus avoided the farmer's scythe. White oaks are among our mightiest trees and can be recognized by their huge, out-reaching limbs, as thick as most tree trunks, and their impressively broad, slightly domed canopies.

Sweet birches have their charms, too. In youth, their bark is beautiful—very tight, dark, and shiny. My younger brother and I discovered that if you chewed a young twig from one of the many seedlings growing beneath the mature trees, it tasted strongly of wintergreen. In the fall, the small, polished leaves turn a lovely shade of yellow, and in the winter, seeds from their abundant catkins cover the snow like millions of little bird tracks.

In the Northeast and in many other parts of the country, homes of all ages are surrounded by the remains of second-growth woodland. So all the delights of the forest are available to anyone with a scrap of wooded land. Free for the looking are the wonderful fall colors and in the winter, the patterns of bare branches against the sky. Woodland attracts dozens of creatures, large and small, and many different kinds of birds. And it can all become an extension of your garden. If the wooded land is yours, you can create a path among the trees. It doesn't have to be long.

In her Newtown garden, Martha McKeon made a delightful little woodland walk with stepping-stones that circle around a couple of trees down by her brook. I gave her water-loving primroses, and she planted hellebores, ferns, and early spring bulbs. The flat fieldstones keep your feet dry and slow your steps so that you can really appreciate the plants beside the path.

At the edge of her woodland, Mary Ann McGourty has

added a few native shrubs—yellow-fruited winterberry and black-haw viburnum, both beloved by avian residents of the forest. On the trunk of a large oak, she plans to grow a rooted layer from the climbing hydrangea she left behind at Hillside Gardens, and she's thinking about naturalizing daffodils among the trees. "I debated about introducing cultivated plants," she says. "Then I thought, well, they are all things that can take care of themselves."

Inspired by Mary Ann's example, I have begun working on a new project. Eventually it will create an extension of the garden that will be beautiful and require no attention whatsoever. Daffodils are the secret. To digress briefly, when I began planting daffodils in the field, my helper was our first Jack Russell terrier puppy. It was slow going. Besides the difficulty of digging into the rough, rocky hillside, I had to keep an eye on Abby.

Suddenly a doe bounded through the field behind us. For a second the puppy froze, and then she was off like a shot. Being fleet of foot in those days, I managed to catch her, but that was the end of daffodil planting for the day. Every year since, I have added to the planting, but last fall Erica did most of the work, putting in about a dozen new clumps, with six or seven bulbs in each hole. It was wonderful in April! Looking out over the top of the computer across the unkempt garden, all I could see was waves of daffodils sweeping farther and farther up the hillside.

Since that single doe dashed past Abby almost thirty years ago, the deer population has exploded, and the forest shelters an expanding herd. The fence only keeps them out of the garden, leaving them access to the field, but they don't touch daffodils. So once planted, these hardy bulbs require no protection and no care. This spring, Erica dug a few more clumps from the most flourishing patches to plant in the empty spaces we would be unable to identify in the fall.

The new daffodil project involves a part of the field that proved too steep and rocky to mow. Tree seedlings colonized the slope and have now become strong saplings and young trees. I'm going to have them thinned out, and then we can start a new planting of daffodils among the trees. In time, I will have a care-free new woodland garden that I can see without setting a foot out of doors.

Every year, the surrounding forest means more to me. In the summer, sunbeams spangle the brown, leaf-littered floor with patches of gold. In the winter, the repetition of straight black tree trunks draws the eye deep into the woods. And with the leaves gone, the sky expands overhead. The view from my windows is completely satisfying, and I don't have to do anything to it. I just sit at the kitchen table or gaze down from my office window and drink it all in. When I do, I don't even notice the imperfections in the garden.

While not everybody is lucky enough to have this particular view, there are other ways to take the eye out of the middle ground and into the distance. Years ago, when I was working with my friend Betty Ajay, we designed a small city garden in New Haven. The long, narrow lot was empty except for trash, but the neighboring brownstones had beautiful old trees in their yards. So we made their trees part of the view we created.

Last fall, in Charlotte, North Carolina, I met a clever local gardener who borrowed her view from a nearby golf course. She opened a "window" in the shrubbery enclosing her garden and framed the rolling greens of the golf course and a tree-covered knoll in the distance. Making the most of a distant prospect and relaxing your hold on the garden can go a long way toward simplifying your life.

❊ GLEANINGS ❊

❊ The world around you

The landscape around me is wooded, and my borrowed view is of trees, thousands of them, that make up the eight-hundred-acre Paugussett State Forest. While the trees belong to the state, the view is mine.

Your landscape may be very different from mine, but there will be something worth looking at. The view from a garden in New York City might offer a tracery of fire escapes against a sliver of open sky. If you live in the suburbs, your view will probably include other houses, backyards, and gardens. If so, there may be part of a neighbor's landscape that could serve as your view. Borrow whatever you need from your neighborhood and surroundings.

❊ A garden and its setting

My garden took shape the way it did because of its setting. Working within that frame, I tried to make the plantings fit into the natural landscape. If I didn't maintain it, the garden would eventually return to its place in the woods. First weeds, then eventually trees would overwhelm the perennials. For a time, a few tough native perennials and some of the daylilies would bring color to a clearing in the forest.

I try to remember this when the garden looks a shambles and comfort myself by looking into the forest. The trees are beautiful, individually and collectively. They gave me pleasure before I even began making the garden, and they give me even more pleasure now.

❋ Making use of your surroundings

If you own even a scrap of woodland, you can make it an extension of your garden by edging it with a few berried and flowering shrubs, as Mary Ann McGourty has done.

Mary Ann simply planted winterberry and viburnum at the edge of her wooded property and plans to naturalize daffodils on the forest floor. But there are a lot of different ways to use your surroundings. A buffer of woodland can belong to your neighbors and yet provide an excellent backdrop for a shrub border, which is the case in Terence Farrell's garden.

When I was working with my friend Betty Ajay, we designed a city garden in downtown New Haven. The lot was very small and narrow, with nothing in it except rubbish. But the neighboring yards boasted beautiful old trees, which we adopted and incorporated into our plan as a background for broadleaf evergreens and flowering shrubs.

A North Carolina gardener whom I met recently employed another device to make use of borrowed landscape. She cut a window in the shrub border enclosing her garden and framed a view of the adjacent golf course with a wooded knoll in the distance.

Drawing attention to a pleasing prospect in the distance can relieve the pressure of garden maintenance and allow you to relax and enjoy the view.

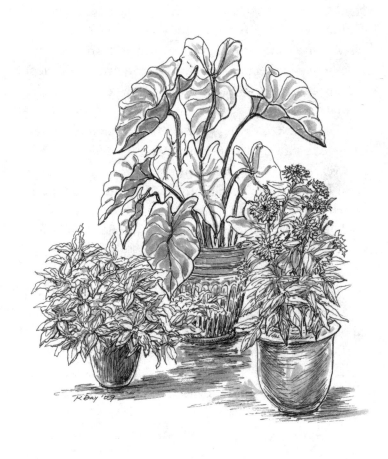

14

Container Gardening:
Arranging Potted Plants with a Purpose

MY INTEREST IN container gardening goes back a long way to the summer of 1949, which I spent with my grandmother and aunt in England. It was Aunt Joan who sowed the seeds of my enduring love of gardens and gardening.

Her own garden was wonderful, but it seemed to me that everywhere I went that summer there were wonderful gardens. I used to hang out of railway carriage windows as the train crept through poor neighborhoods in different cities, to admire the tiny backyard gardens grown almost entirely in rusty tin cans, old washtubs, and other makeshift containers.

The row houses were crammed together and their backyards paved, but that didn't stop their owners from gardening. Nasturtiums in window boxes trailed down and over the pavement, and climbing roses smothered shabby walls. Some homeowners also kept chickens and grew peas and broad beans against their henhouses.

It was a great lesson in what can be done to make the smallest, most unpromising site into a garden. And though it would be many years before I would do any container gardening myself, the memory of those backyards along the railway tracks remained with me.

The eleven years between my first trip to England and my marriage to Martin were busy and peripatetic, but once we had a house of our own I instinctively began gardening. My early attempts resulted in naïve copies of my aunt's perennial borders. As I gradually got the hang of it, the borders became more and more complex, a trend that would continue for the next forty years. In the meantime I also rediscovered container gardening.

It began as a practical tool for teaching a class at the New York Botanical Garden called "Color for Gardeners." If you are going to talk about color combinations, you need to be able to show them. I didn't have all the necessary colors in the perennial borders, so I began scouring the local nurseries for annuals to pot up and arrange together to illustrate different color schemes. In the process, I discovered how much fun it was to plan the colors, find the right plants, plant them, and then set out the pots in attractive groupings on the terrace.

However, the terrace did not come together as a garden until a chance meeting with a group of impressively knowledgeable younger gardeners, who led me to Peter Wooster's garden. The year was 1989, and tender perennials were beginning to be "hot." My delightful new friends drew me into the heady world of exotic plants from South America, South Africa, Australia, and New Zealand. As these younger gardeners and their colleagues, along with their eager clients, launched the gardening boom of the 1990s, I happily jumped aboard.

Peter and his gardener, Gary Keim, deployed tender perennials in novel and unexpected ways. They used them in containers set on tall bases as focal points and to add drama to mixed borders among the hardy perennials, shrubs, and ornamental trees. In one small specialized bed, Peter put a new spin on a Victorian bedding scheme by using the latest cultivars of coleus and cannas in a circular pattern around a potted banana plant that dominated the bed.

Having never before been a fan of either coleus or cannas, I went overboard for the new foliage colors and patterns in coleus and for the expanded color range of the canna flowers—yellow, orange, and pink. These large, eye-catching plants quickly became the stars of my own containers.

But of all the dazzling plants I met thanks to Peter, my hands-down favorite remains *Brugmansia* 'Charles Grimaldi'. Peter gave me a cutting that summer, which I grew indoors over the winter and moved outside in the spring, and I have taken cuttings ever since. As I write, those taken last October are out on the terrace in six-inch pots, awaiting the move to bigger pots before finally becoming the "trees" in this year's container garden.

In their native South America, brugmansias really do grow into trees, but in pots mine reach only about six feet. Nevertheless, the growth spurt is amazing when you consider their small size at the beginning of the summer. That's only part of the brugmansia's allure. The blossoms, shaped like downward-hanging trumpets, are a foot long and the most delicious shade of pale yellow, aging to an even more delicious shade of apricot. In the evening, the heavy sweetness of their perfume evokes languorous nights of tropical splendor.

The color experiments in pots put me a step nearer the creation of a container garden, and the infusion of large, dramatic specimens like the brugmansias and cannas put me over the top. Having been the set designer for innumerable summer stock and student theatrical productions, I suddenly realized that making a container garden on the terrace was very similar to designing a set for the stage.

In summer stock, the trick was to create a different set every week—on a shoestring and at the double. Of necessity, the means were simple. The crew and I shuffled the props and set pieces around and slapped on a new coat of paint. I found this technique worked equally well on the terrace and began rearranging the pots every year, using different plants and painting our little wrought metal table and four chairs a different color. Voila! Another opening of another show . . .

I soon discovered other similarities between set design and making container gardens. In the theater, doorways and other openings are important because they create a sense of expectation. The same is true of a garden gate or an entrance arch covered with vines. Partial concealment heightens the feeling of anticipation. Yet the visitor is never in doubt about the way into the garden.

I use a lattice archway at one end of the terrace to dramatize the entrance to the container garden and to create a bit of mystery. At the same time, the arch provides height and a surface on which to grow different vines every year. Vertical gardening using arches, trellises, and obelisks is a practical way to increase the gardening possibilities of any small space, whether deck, patio, or city rooftop.

Before the days of the container garden, Martin and I were never very happy about our terrace, though we improved it in 1980 by replacing the broken concrete slabs, which were a danger to

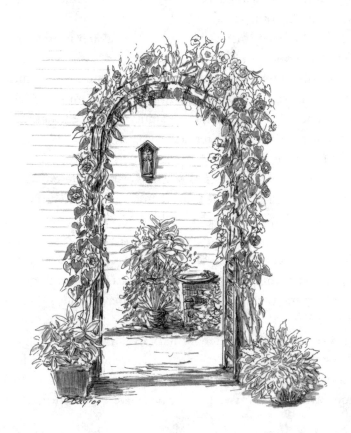

life and limb. We would have liked flagstone, but it proved too expensive, so we settled for another concrete slab. And as an after-thought enclosed it with a low brick wall capped with flagstone.

Although the wall never served its original purpose as extra seating, it was perfect for staging potted plants. Eventually the containers became so numerous that they completely enclosed the terrace, creating a "garden room" with leafy walls and "window" openings through which to look out at the rest of the garden. A sense of enclosure is important in a garden, and it's easy using plants in containers. You can make a wall of potted plants as dense or as open as you like and wherever you like or need a partition.

A stage and a terrace or deck have a lot more in common than you might think. Their dimensions are fixed and predetermined by the architecture of which they are a part. You can divide up the space in different ways with walls of wood and muslin or ranks of potted plants, but you are ultimately limited to the size of the set or garden. As these relatively small spaces are intended for use, traffic patterns become an issue.

In the theater, you have an obligation to the director, who will determine where and how the actors move around the stage. So the set designer's first job is to make getting around safe and easy for them. The same is true in the garden. Paths should guide visitors safely and efficiently to their destination. Therefore, I usually make a path down the long dimension of the container garden to provide access to the dining area at the far end.

This axial path intersects with a shorter, broader path from the sliding doors in the kitchen to the widest opening in the low brick wall. The center opening, leading into the garden proper, offers a view of the upper lawn and perennial borders, and glimpses of the field beyond the old stone wall.

Framing this view is always the first step in assembling the container garden. I begin by planting the two big pots that will flank the opening. It is important to employ specimens that are tall enough and full enough to keep the onlooker's eye from roaming across the whole landscape at once. A frame controls your attention and heightens awareness of whatever lies within its boundaries.

As most container gardens are closely related to the architecture of a house or other building, they are dominated by materials with hard surfaces, straight lines, and sharp corners. Inside corners pinch the space they enclose, and outside corners thrust their intrusive sharpness into the natural world. Plants can help reconcile the angularity of architecture with the softness and curving lines of the natural landscape.

For example, a small upright tree tucked into an inside corner can bring that tight, uninteresting space to life and create a link between house and garden. Trailing plants do something similar for the sharp edges of pots and window boxes, while climbers like morning glories and their many kin can be used to drape an ugly chain-link fence or smother a panel of lattice in order to hide an eyesore, like our dog run.

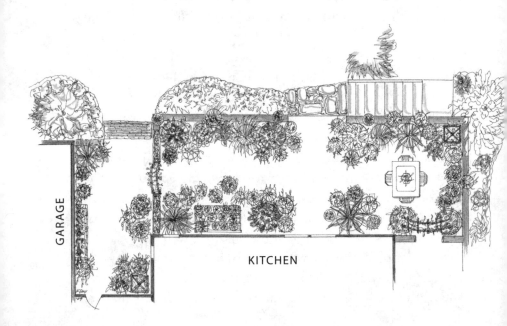

In about 1800, when our house was built, most dwellings were a reasonable size and had a pleasing balance between wall space and openings for doors and windows. But today comfort and convenience often trump aesthetic considerations. We wanted an attached garage and a covered breezeway leading to the kitchen.

A garage is seldom a pretty sight, and ours had one particularly unattractive blank wall adjacent to the terrace. To take the curse off the wall, Martin planted a little pear tree against it in a well made in the concrete. Over time, he pruned the pear into a creditable espalier, which now covers two-thirds of the garage wall. Divided into smaller segments by the leafy branches of the tree, the monotonous pattern of the siding has become much less obtrusive.

The north wall of our kitchen presents a similar problem, a lot of siding uninterrupted except by the sliding doors and a couple of small, oddly placed windows. But in the summer, the container garden with its massive brugmansias and jungle of other tropical plants hides the rest of the kitchen wall anyway.

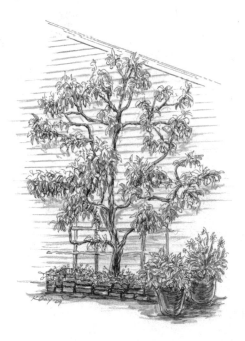

Although container gardens can serve practical purposes, for me they have mostly been for fun, combining my love of theater and of gardening and permitting me to grow more new and different plants in a single summer than I could possibly grow in the ground. I've also gotten a tremendous kick out of surprising friends with wild new color schemes every year.

The container gardens have had to take a back seat to the perennial borders for the last four years, but it's a cheering thought that with a little help transporting bags of potting soil to the terrace and moving the heavy pots, I can go on gardening into advanced old age. Container gardening requires a fraction of the physical work that an in-the-ground garden demands and provides much of the same joy and satisfaction.

✤ GLEANINGS ✤

❈ Early warning signs

Even as a seventeen-year-old visitor to England, I was intrigued by paved backyards in London filled with plants
in makeshift containers. While a container garden of my
own was a long way off, clearly I had leanings in that
direction.

❈ Beginning a container garden

Quite by chance in the mid-eighties, I needed to photo-
graph specific color combinations for a class I was teaching. I went to a couple of nurseries, bought plants, potted
them up, and arranged different color schemes on the terrace. The assembled pots served their purpose and looked
so attractive that the next year there were more pots, and
before I knew it I was hooked.

If you think gardening in containers might appeal to
you, take a ride to the nearest nursery and stock up on
pots of different sizes—including a few large ones for big
plants like cannas. For me, the leap from collection of
potted plants to garden came after I was introduced to
some of the new canna cultivars, like 'Tropicana' with its
vividly striped leaves.

I fell in love with these and other flamboyant tropicals
that became the building blocks of my container gardens.
They will be invaluable to you, too. Huge plants like the
brugmansias from South America become the trees in
your potted garden; statuesque cannas, the shrubs; and
trailing sweet potato vines, the ground covers.

Being able to keep some of the tender plants over the

winter gave me an idea. By potting them up again in the spring, rearranging them on the terrace, and adding annuals and a few new tropicals, I could have a different garden and a different color scheme every year. To a former set designer it was irresistible, and painting the metal furniture to match was the finishing touch.

✤ Arranging potted plants with a purpose

There are striking similarities between set design and making a garden with potted plants. Doorways and arched openings are to drawing room comedies what gates and archways are to gardens. They whet your appetite for surprises and provide access.

So start with the doorway to your house. The addition of potted plants on either side makes it welcoming. Or place a lattice archway at the access point of your patio and plant vines in pots on either side. The vine-covered archway offers an invitation to enter but hides part of the garden beyond. Partial concealment creates a bit of mystery.

Our terrace already has a gardenlike sense of enclosure because the slab of concrete is surrounded by a low brick wall, but you can create walls with potted plants anywhere you want them. To frame a view or hide an eyesore, use statuesque plants like cannas or tall dahlias and bushy coleus.

Controlling traffic is as important in a garden as it is on stage. So you will need to suggest a route through your container garden. Mine has a broad path from the sliding doors in the kitchen to the wide opening in the wall, and a narrow path from the entrance archway to a small dining area at the far end of the terrace.

Turning a terrace into a garden means softening the hard edges and surfaces of man-made architecture with the pliant forms of plants. And breaking up blank walls with evergreens in pots, vines on a lattice panel, or large, leafy plants like brugmansias, which have the height and spread of small trees.

❧ All of the pleasure for a fraction of the work

The means may be theatrical, but there is nothing fake about a container garden. It is the real thing. And for anyone who can't do the heavy labor of in-the-ground gardening, gardening in containers can provide much of the same pleasure.

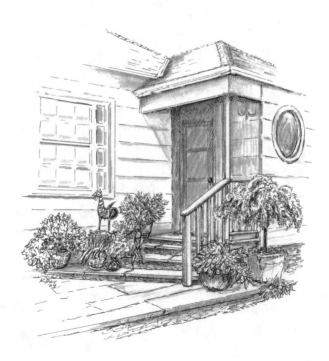

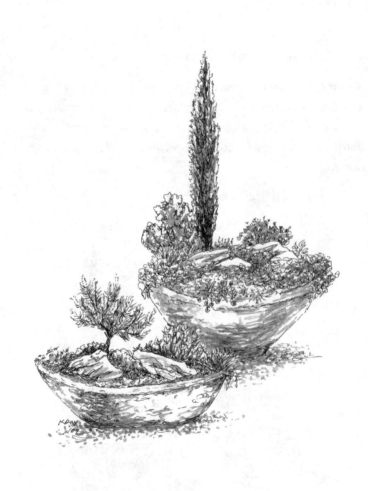

15

Miniature Landscapes:
Exploring New Ways to Garden

MUCH HAS CHANGED since I began writing this book. Last fall ended gently, and a harsh but comparatively snowless winter followed. The eagerly awaited spring has been cool, damp, and blissfully drawn out over many weeks—more beautiful than anything I can ever remember. The rhododendrons left me speechless. So spectacular were they that a perfect stranger, walking in the state forest, stopped to ask if he could bring his wife to see them. Now 'Boule de Neige', the white-flowered one in front, is losing its blossoms, and 'Scintillation', the crème de la crème of pinks, is fading fast. Summer is in sight.

While all this has been happening in the garden, my body has been doing a ten-year-fast-forward to advanced old age, and the hip complaint of March has become the problem to be solved sometime this summer. For all intents and purposes, I have been unable to garden for nearly two months, leaving Erica with her hands full. But she has more than risen to the occasion, and the faithful Terence has stepped in and taken up the slack.

While I am very much dismayed by my limitations, I know I'm not alone. Sooner or later, every older gardener faces a similar challenge. At some point, we all find ourselves asking, "If I can't get out there and dig, plant, and prune as I used to do, *what am I going to do?*"

I still don't know the answer, but for anyone who loves plants and planting enough to keep trying new things, there are other ways to garden. If you are what Lori Chips, manager of the alpine department at Oliver Nurseries in Fairfield, Connecticut, calls a "plant geek," you might be interested in making miniature landscapes in hypertufa troughs. She describes this form of gardening as "just a load of fun," and her enthusiasm is irresistible.

The idea of trough gardening has a long, distinguished history. Like many horticultural traditions, it began in England. British plant hunter and writer Reginald Farrer is credited with introducing gardeners to alpine plants and to the art of rock gardening in the early years of the twentieth century.

In 1979, I joined the North American Rock Garden Society—then simply the American Rock Garden Society—and soon discovered that my easygoing style of perennial gardening was a world apart from the exacting art of rock gardening. Plants adapted to the inhospitable environment of the mountains have very specific requirements. Serious rock gardeners spend a lifetime studying their habitats and a fortune visiting them to learn more about growing these beautiful but willful little plants.

In England, alpines used to be grown in specially constructed rockeries or in the old stone troughs once used to water livestock. Filled with the kind of gravely, fast-draining soil favored by denizens of the high country, stone drinking troughs provided alpine enthusiasts with a natural-looking container suitable for rock gardening. By embedding realistically tilted pieces of rock in the soil and adding plants properly scaled to the small world of the trough, they created believable miniature landscapes.

When British rock gardeners eventually ran out of old stone troughs, they came up with an ingenious solution—troughs made from hypertufa, a mixture of cement, peat moss, and perlite. Tufa is a calcareous rock formed in the mineral-rich water of mountain streams. Porous and pockmarked with holes, it allows water to seep through it.

Like tufa, the hypertufa mixture hardens into a rocklike substance that is permeable, allowing excess water to escape through the walls of the trough. Good drainage is a must for alpine plants. As Lori Chips puts it, "The issue with alpines is drainage.

For real estate agents it may be location, location, location, but for alpines it's drainage, drainage, drainage, and soil." Alpines are used to living on the lean side in a mix of rock particles of different sizes.

While they thrive on this spare diet, most remain small—smaller than a baby's clenched fist and often dome-shaped. Rock gardeners call this form a "cushion" or a "bun." And Lori can tell you why these little plants assume such a low profile. First, it's to withstand the constant battering of gale-force winds, ever present at high altitudes. The foliage of taller plants would be torn to shreds, but alpines crouch down and pack their minute leaves tightly around them.

Another hazard of life at the top is the showers of pebbles and broken rock dislodged by wind, rain, and snow that hurtle down from above. The half-dome shape with its sloping sides shrugs off moving debris, allowing it to roll up, over, and off the plant. There is something about the diminutive size of alpine plants pitted against the elements that arouses protective feelings among susceptible gardeners. And the sight of a perfect little hemisphere of saxifrage brings them to their knees. Lori attributes this reaction to the "cuteness factor."

But you don't have to climb a mountain in order to experi-

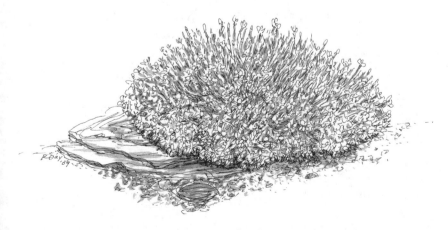

ence the cuteness factor in small plants. The Northeast boasts spring wildflowers that have the same effect. If you have ever bent over a tiny tuft of bluettes in the woods and gurgled, "Oh, how cute!" you may easily become attracted to alpine plants and trough gardening. Trough gardening allows adults to play with little plants and to create miniature landscapes and gardens without feeling foolish.

Although hypertufa troughs are specifically intended to keep the fussier little mountain dwellers happy, there is no hard-and-fast rule about what to grow in them. You could fill a trough with ordinary potting soil and try any small plants that take your fancy. However, if you'd like to try simple rock gardening, there are easy alpines, like dianthus, creeping phlox, sedums, and of course, bulletproof hens-and-chicks. Hens-and-chicks are my speed, though I've also had a little campanula growing in one of my troughs for many years.

Like any garden, a trough garden should offer the eye an interesting tour of different sizes, shapes, and textures. It should also have a bit of structure. You need something vertical to anchor your miniature garden and something rounded to provide contrast; something low to knit the rocks and plants together, and something trailing to soften the edge of the trough.

Your miniature landscape represents a larger landscape; therefore, the rocks and plants should be believable in terms of their relative sizes. For instance, if your highest tree is 10 inches tall and finely textured, the ground cover should have suitably small, delicate leaves.

For the vertical element in your Lilliputian landscape, Lori recommends a dwarf conifer like the tiny Alberta spruce *Picea glauca* 'Jean's Dilly', named for Jean Iseli from Iseli Nursery in Oregon; and for rounded shapes, a couple of dear little mugo pines, as plump and prickly as baby hedgehogs—'Paul's Dwarf' and 'Donna's Mini'. Two miniature cultivars of our native hemlock—*Tsuga canadensis* 'Minuta' and 'Cole's Prostrate'—are also suitable for trough gardens. 'Cole's Prostrate' remains low and spreading and 'Minuta', according to the Oliver Nurseries catalog, eventually becomes a globe the size of a bowling ball.

Oliver Nurseries has been a source of dwarf conifers, alpine plants, and hypertufa troughs since the early seventies. At that time, John Oliver, founder of the nursery, hired Ellie Brinkerhoff Spingarn to head the new alpine department. Ellie had already been awarded every honor the American Rock Garden Society could bestow upon her. Kim Proctor, who worked with her, said, "She opened up a whole new world to everybody at the nursery and to Fairfield County."

Today, Lori Chips carries the torch, and the alpine department is thriving. You can get ideas for miniature gardens from a charming display of planted troughs in every imaginable size and shape set on top of a handsome stone retaining wall. But you don't need a stone wall. Troughs can also be used on doorsteps and patios or tucked into the front borders.

The flora of the mountains is intriguing, and you may get caught up in the excitement, especially if you join the North American Rock Garden Society. But the point here is that trough gardens are easy to maintain. Lori says, "Weeding will take you about five minutes—not hours. You do a bit of pruning here and pinching there, top-dress your trough with a handful of grit once a year, and you're done." The purpose of the grit covering— I use gravel—is to keep the soil underneath cool and moist and the leaves of the alpines dry.

It is no wonder that Oliver Nurseries looms large in this chapter. I have been a regular visitor to the nursery since the mid-seventies, and Kim Proctor grew up there. In 1973 her mother married John Oliver, and Kim began her career in horticulture. She worked at the nursery during school and college vacations and full time for the next fifteen years, with a hiatus here and there to raise children and design gardens.

In her spare time and purely for her own pleasure, she has

made gardens of all kinds, from meadows to troughs to bonsai, a fascinating way to garden on the smallest possible scale. Although she protests that she is not a bonsai expert, Kim's collection of miniature trees suggests otherwise. They look as real as anything growing in nature, only much, much smaller. This is the essence of bonsai. The miniature trees must look completely natural.

Ignorant as I was about bonsai, I found myself very moved by an exhibition at the Chicago Botanic Garden last year. Having heretofore belonged to the school of thought that plants should be allowed to mature into their natural shapes with a bit of tweaking here and there, I had never really appreciated this living art form. But these plants caught my attention and stirred my soul.

While their beauty was inspiring, it was their evocation of mature, even ancient trees, perfect in every respect—from thick, twisted trunks to gnarled, wide-reaching branches—that made such a profound impression. The shallow bonsai pots rested on invisible metal grids above a sheet of water, and behind them semitranslucent panels hung from the ceiling. The entire exhibit seemed to float in space, and the effect took my breath away.

As Japanese gardeners understand bonsai, an art form they adopted from China, it is about shaping nature to manifest its essence. They believe that human beings should work with plants to reveal nature's ideal form, while Western gardeners tend to shear and prune to make nature conform to *their* ideal.

In his introduction to *The Essentials of Bonsai* (Timber Press, 1982), Donald Richie explains just what bonsai is all about: "It is, precisely, a microcosm, containing within it, unchanged in everything but size, the mystery of the universe." To this special form of garden making, Kim brings the eyes of an artist, the skills of a horticulturist, an open mind, and a deep feeling for nature.

In her collection, a little white azalea, on the verge of flowering when I last saw it, is her oldest bonsai—about fifteen years old. Left to its own devices, this small member of the rhododendron family would eventually achieve a height of two feet or more instead of just a few inches. Kim says that some people would say that she was cheating by starting with such a small plant in the first place. "In true bonsai," she says, "there are ancient trident maples, hornbeams, and other trees that in the ground would reach fifty or sixty feet."

The art of training miniature trees came from East to West in the person of Yugi Yoshimura, considered the father of popular bonsai in the non-Asian world. In 1960 he gave a lecture in New York attended by a spellbound John Oliver. Returning to his nursery, Oliver set about finding a bone fide expert in bonsai to head a new department and teach classes. While Kim's interest had been piqued at that time, her life took off in other directions and she soon became too busy with kids and work. "It really has only been within the last six or seven years that I've gotten involved again," she says. "But I've really enjoyed it. I love

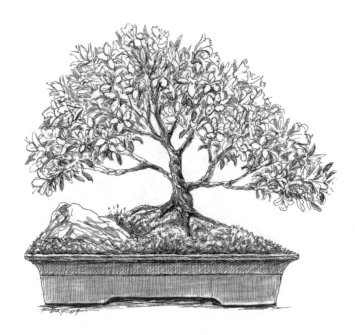

the different plants and the different pots and setting up these miniature landscapes with rocks and mosses."

On a recent visit, she showed me a beautiful little maple, *Acer palmatum* 'Otome-zakura'. The roots, growing over a wonderfully craggy-looking small rock, were partly exposed and twisted, giving the effect of great age. So I was amazed when Kim said, "Oh, no, I just potted that. It's one of the flowering maples, so-called because the spring growth is so showy. When the leaves first come out, they are the deepest, purest cherry red. Then they fade to a bronze-green. By midsummer they become almost green, and in the fall they turn an orangey red.

"Actually, Ross got the flowering maple two or three years ago from Mountain Maples. I wintered it over in the hoop house because the flowering maples are not as hardy as other Japanese maples around here. I only potted it up this spring. The pot is a classic bonsai pot, which measures fourteen inches long, ten

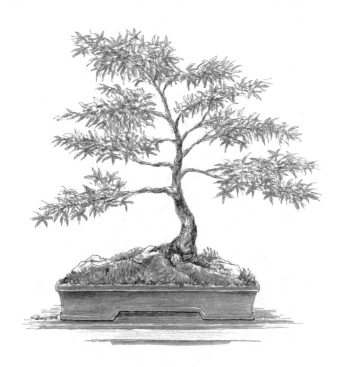

inches wide, and three inches deep." Traditionally, bonsai pots are either oval or rectangular and surprisingly shallow. The rule is that the depth of the pot should approximate the girth of the tree trunk.

Kim showed me quite a large weeping juniper in another large but much deeper pot. "You can start trees out in these bigger pots after you've trimmed down their roots. You let them get acclimated to this size—twelve inches high by fifteen inches across—and give them time to get used to the idea of thinking smaller. After a year or two, you prune the roots and get them into bonsai pots, which are less than half as deep but just about as wide.

"At this point, the weeping juniper is just a potted tree. For it to become a true bonsai, I'd have to spend the next four or five or six years taking it out of this pot and pruning the roots, and eventually working it back into a smaller pot. But it already has a terrific shape, nice exfoliating bark, and some really nice age to it."

Kim loves her miniature trees and claims that their maintenance is not too exacting. During the summer she waters them daily. "When I get home in the afternoon, I walk around with the hose on a light spray and wait until I see water coming out of the bottom of the pots. Then I just wander around asking, 'How are you?' and 'How are you?' and 'How are you?'

"Because the bonsai are in such shallow pots, they can dry out quickly, but having them close to the back of the house, where we come and go every day, reminds me to water them. And underneath this big maple, they get plenty of protection from the hot sun."

While Kim admits that there is a lot to learn about bonsai, one thing that gardeners have when they get "some really nice age" to them is time. And to make a study of this absorbing, thought-provoking form of gardening would be time well spent.

❧ GLEANINGS ❧

❧ Rock gardening

Rock gardening simply means creating a garden with alpine plants, and take it from Lori Chips, manager of the alpine department at Oliver Nurseries—it's fun. Although alpine enthusiasts lust after challenging jewels that come from inaccessible places and resist taming, there are plenty of easier alpines for the rest of us to grow.

❧ The nature of alpine plants

Alpine plants appear to have been tailor-made for miniature gardens, but they are in fact nature-made to survive harsh climates. Their leaves tend to be small and tightly packed; otherwise they would be torn to shreds by the winds that constantly batter mountain peaks.

At lower altitudes, some of the choicest plants become cranky because they can't tolerate humidity or poor drainage. But growing them in a gritty soil in permeable hypertufa troughs goes a long way toward keeping them happy. And making alpine gardens in troughs goes a long way toward keeping adventurous gardeners happy with a minimum of physical effort.

In the same way that antique dollhouses replicate period homes, a trough garden suggests a natural landscape and should be credible in terms of scale and proportion. There are wonderful little plants to do the job: minute hemlocks, dwarf Alberta spruces less than a foot high, tight little "cushion" plants, and tiny creeping ground covers.

❧ Getting started with alpines

The best way to get started with alpines and trough gardens is to read H. Lincoln Foster's *Rock Gardening: A Guide to Growing Alpines and Other Wildflowers in American Gardens* (Houghton Mifflin, 1968). It's a treat to read, and even contains a recipe for hypertufa that you can mix up in your garage. Copies, used and new, are still available online at www.amazon.com. Also worth looking at is *The Rock Garden Plant Primer: Easy, Small Plants for Containers, Patios, and the Open Garden* by Christopher Grey-Wilson (Timber, 2009).

Another good way to learn about rock gardening is to join the North American Rock Garden Society. You can find a membership form online at www.nargs.org. And if you live in Connecticut, the display of planted hypertufa troughs at Oliver Nurseries in Fairfield will inspire you.

❧ Bonsai, the art and craft of growing miniature trees

Ever since I saw a remarkable exhibition of bonsai at the Chicago Botanic Garden, my mind has repeatedly wandered back to these exquisite miniature trees. Although a joint venture between humans and nature, bonsai involves the human being only in the un-self-conscious role of revealing the essence of the tree. Each tree must remain completely faithful to nature and appear as true to itself as if it were still growing in the wild. Only its tiny size separates the miniature tree from its real nature.

Bonsai was adopted from China by the Japanese about twelve hundred years ago and had never been seen in Europe until the twentieth century. It arrived at Oliver

Nurseries in 1960 after founder John Oliver heard Yugi Yoshimura, the father of popular bonsai, speak in New York. Kim Proctor became intrigued while she was working at Oliver Nurseries.

�֍ A gardener's collection of bonsai

Although she insists that she is not a bonsai expert, Kim has grown a fascinating and beautiful collection of tiny trees in the shallow vessels decreed suitable by classical bonsai experts. While Kim doesn't follow every rule of classical bonsai, she has learned how to gradually acclimate trees and shrubs to culture in the confines of a classic bonsai pot. By root pruning and repotting the tree or shrub over a period of a few years into smaller and smaller containers, she persuades plants whose natural dimensions might be measured in feet to remain small and grow happily to a size measured in inches.

The art of bonsai appeals on an intellectual and emotional level to artistic gardeners who are attentive to line, form, and balance. According to Kim, maintenance isn't as exacting as one might think, but the style of gardening does demand vigilance about watering because the shallow containers dry up very quickly.

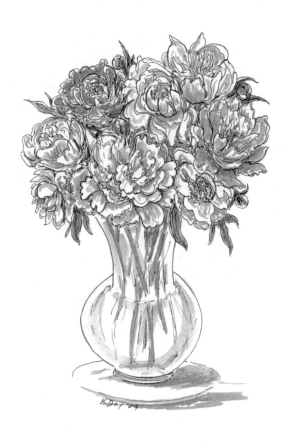

16

A Summing Up:
Making the Most of What You Have Left

LAST NIGHT AFTER a day of rain, I cut the last of the late peonies, the ones Erica had spared from the week before. We were washed out this week. But the garden, shaggy as it is, still makes me very happy. In the strange underwater light of a misty, overcast June morning, it seems to hum and vibrate with vivid yellow-greens.

Martin always wanted a honey locust (*Gleditsia triacanthos*) with bright chartreuse new growth, like the ones he saw in the grocery store parking lot. But with a little persuasion, he settled instead for a golden black locust (*Robinia pseudoacacia* 'Frisia'), which holds its bright color all season. The honey locusts turn green by early summer. Although he chided me for not allowing him to choose his own tree, he loved 'Frisia', which is at its glowing best right now.

Once the blossoms of the rhododendrons have fallen and the irises and peonies have finished flowering, the garden is entirely green. The greens are wonderful in mid-June, especially after a rain. Every shade and tint between almost yellow and almost blue is represented. At the bright end of the spectrum, there are the sharp yellow-greens of the spireas and the locust, and the mellow golds of the false cypresses; and at the opposite end, soothing tints of blue among the various dwarf spruces, and of course the fresh midgreens of youthful maple leaves against the much darker greens of the forest background.

My friend Betty Ajay, a gifted and successful landscape designer for half a century who died last year, would approve of my

189

garden at the moment. I was an enormous fan of Betty's work and was her assistant for about eighteen months in the mid-eighties before I began writing seriously. I learned a lot from Betty, especially about the use of space, but we were poles apart in our color preferences. Mine were for hot colors, hers for cool greens. In my ignorance, I thought green gardens lovely but not exciting enough. I was still intoxicated by flowers and the lively, knock-your-socks-off effects of high contrast. But like so many other things, my view of green gardens has changed.

Now I love nothing more than this green phase in my own garden before the onslaught of the daylilies. While I have always thrilled to their trumpet calls of red, orange, yellow, and gold, the thought of all that demanding color now makes me a little tired. I feel like Maurice Chevalier in *Gigi* who at an advanced age wistfully asks his former mistress, "Am I getting old?" To which she tactfully replies, "Not you."

Well, maybe Maurice Chevalier's character is not, but I am getting old, and that's why I am writing this book—to blaze a trail for other gardeners to follow or not, as they choose, but to show them that there is a way to continue gardening into a ripe old age. For the trailblazer the way has not proven easy, but the words of a gardening friend whom I admire have kept me going.

After a recent visit in early May, Rita Buchanan—you met Rita in Chapter 10—sent me a note that I will always keep. She wrote: "Outside, your garden is now rich with mature plants, broad and mounded; you've simplified it so that the plants have plenty of space and are not at all crowded or cluttered. It seems calm to me. What do you think Betty Ajay would say?"

Because I have always valued both Rita's and Betty's opinions, these words gave me heart. But it was the next paragraph that got me over the hump of a writer's block. She said that it was important for me to be writing this book. "You've been wrestling with the ideas for as long as I've known you! Now at last you're ready to say what you've learned about it all."

What have I learned about it all? I have just hung up the phone after talking to Terence Farrell, who transplanted an enkianthus from my garden to his last Sunday. He reports that the shrub has settled in nicely and is already putting out new growth.

It is not an ideal time to transplant shrubs, but having read that enkianthus is quite shallow rooted, Terence decided to go for it. This way, he can cosset and water it all summer and will know that it is still alive before it finally drops its colorful foliage in November and goes dormant. Mulched, it should make it through the winter in fine shape.

Watching the development of the Farrell garden has been one of the joys of the last couple of years. The intelligence and passion Terence brings to his garden making thrills and inspires

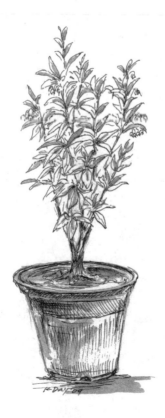

me. And I love the way he shares it and includes the twins, now seven years old, in this new and wonderful outdoor activity. His wife, Rosa, has taken enchanting photographs of Terence and Ryan absorbed in their work.

The Farrells are part of the answer to what I've learned about gardening. I see in Terence and his children two more generations of gardeners. And what is so special about being a gardener? Gardeners harbor a longing for beauty and perfection. Because of what they do, they never lose sight of the small but vital place that each individual holds in the great fabric of nature. Being a gardener stops you from the willing destruction of the fragile world on which we all depend for food, health, and the air we breathe. And if gardening doesn't make you a better person, at least it reveals the best that is in you.

If you wonder whether you would like gardening or not, try it and you will quickly find out. You don't need to know anything to start. I didn't. But here is a good test. Do you mind getting dirt under your fingernails? Can you calmly swat away an insect without wanting to flee indoors? Do close encounters with small, wiggling creatures formerly beneath your notice alarm you, or are they a source of interest? Does clearing a weedy patch of no man's land thrill you out of all proportion to the accomplishment? And finally, having cleared the spot and planted something in it, do you step back and smile with pride? If so, you are a gardener.

I have talented friends who design gardens for other people, and I rejoice on their behalf when they find clients interested enough in plants to want a garden. But it makes me even happier to hear that their clients take an active interest in working in their gardens. The designers whose work I like most are those who actively engage their clients in the garden-making process. Kim is such a designer. She has often made converts of her clients and happily collaborates with them in the creation of their dream gardens. Janet Gordon and her garden in Easton, Connecticut, come instantly to mind.

One wet, drizzly morning in May, Kim took me to visit Janet in her mountaintop paradise. Everywhere, rivulets, trickles, and torrents of pink bleeding heart ran down the steep, mossy sides of rock ledges that Janet had uncovered herself. On top of the ledges, wood poppies, Virginia bluebells, and other spring flowers—all in full bloom—grew out of fissures in the rock. Thousands of plants, the vast majority propagated by Janet herself, filled every crack and crevice and carpeted the woodland floor. It was hauntingly beautiful. But the most memorable scene from that morning was of Janet—head to foot in a bright blue slicker—on her hands and knees in the rain, digging plants for Kim and me to take home. That's what I think gardening is all about.

The gardens that touch me most are brought forth from the hearts, minds, and imaginations of their owner-creators and are shaped by their hands—gardens that evolve inch by inch, season by season, decade by decade. The value of this slow development over time is that the gardener learns by looking. And if you look

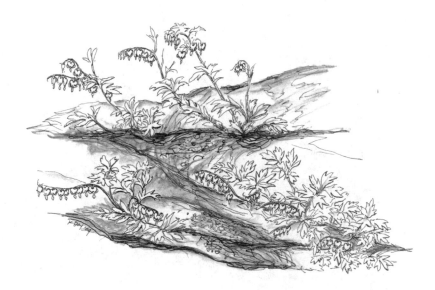

hard enough, you will eventually see. Although seeing takes time and patience, it's worth the effort because from what you have done before, you will *see* what to do next.

Take Terence, for example, who is highly intelligent and has been blessed with an intuitive sense of spatial relationships. He has also learned how to look and is beginning to see his land-scape. He realized that the front walk, which runs parallel to the façade of the house, was too narrow. The house seemed to loom over it. I noticed it immediately. The next time I came, the walk had been doubled in width and looked most inviting. The house seemed to have backed off and now sat comfortably on its site.

Already other areas around the Farrell garden, which is still young as befits its creator and his family, have begun to come together: the beds around the foundations are deep enough and full enough to hold the house in place, while a semicircular shrub border is taking shape around the edge of the sweeping lawn that slopes downward, away from the house. It is exciting to watch Terence wrestling with issues of size—now and later—of the shrubs in relation to a background of second-growth wood-

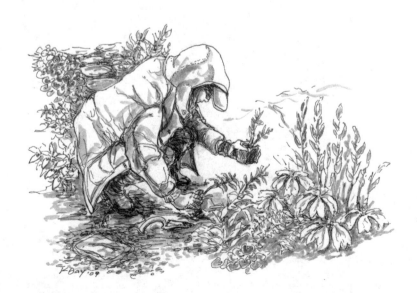

land. I see him learning the way I learned, and it warms the cockles of my heart.

Among the things that I have learned over the years is that a garden must belong to its site. Stanley Kunitz, poet laureate of the United States and winner of numerous poetry awards, was also a passionate gardener. In *The Wild Braid* he talks about his Provincetown, Massachusetts, garden, and you will find in this thin volume more gardening wisdom than in tomes of many thousands of words. He wrote the book when he was approaching one hundred years old. And here is what a poet, lifetime gardener, and artist has to say about the relationship between garden and site: "It is imperative for any gardener to respect the land before alterations, modifications, or plans for the design of the garden are made. If a garden doesn't fit into that landscape and reflect it in some way, it's an invasion, an occupation."

He goes on to say that gardening has many collaborative aspects to it—an idea that I wholeheartedly endorse. Says Kunitz, "You're helping to create a living poem. Philosophically, the garden is a co-creation; it expresses something of the character of the place itself, something that any human intervening there must respect."

Having nature as co-creator allows gardeners to fulfill the yearning many of us feel to be artists. Like painters, gardeners make decisions about size, shape, color, and texture, and like sculptors and architects, we work in three dimensions. Sculptors carve and model solid forms, and architects contain and organize space within structure. Gardeners use structure and form, too. We enclose space that otherwise has no boundaries with walls, fences, or hedges and furnish our enclosures with forms of different sizes and shapes supplied by nature.

There are many parallels between gardening and the arts, but there is also one striking difference. Only the garden is subject to constant change. For the gardener, time is the fourth dimension. Nature gives us the material with which to create a kind of living art and joins with us in the nurture of our plants. But over time, gardeners must provide the patience and determination to ride out the storms, extremes of temperature, and other vicissitudes with which our co-creator tests our mettle. And as always, we have to live with uncertainty.

Certainty in a garden, as in life, is a comforting illusion that lets us bumble along quite happily from day to day until something goes awry. The reality is that change is constant—often slow and subtle, as in the maturation of a maple tree. But sometimes it is swift and brutal, as in the felling of a giant specimen in a hurricane. For this reason and many others, I really believe that gardening is good training for life. Gardeners simply get used to the ebb and flow of the growing seasons, good and bad. Most of us just "keep on keeping on," as Winston Churchill is reputed to have said during the Second World War.

Aging makes keeping on harder, but the story I have pinned on my bulletin board puts it all in perspective. Violinist Itzhak Perlman was crippled by polio in childhood and walks with the aid of braces on his legs and a pair of crutches. At a concert on the night of November 18, 1995, at Avery Fisher Hall in New York City, one of the strings of his violin suddenly snapped during the performance. Stunned, the audience held their collective breath, expecting Perlman to stop and leave the stage. Instead, he paused, then continued playing—adjusting, creating, compensating as he went along, and when he put down his bow at the end of the concert, a mighty roar of applause filled the hall. When it had died down, he spoke to the audience: "You know, sometimes it is the artist's task to find out how much music you can still make with what you have left."

Making the most of what you have left is also the older gardener's task. How beautiful can you make your garden with the resources you still have at your command? This is the question I keep asking myself. I don't have the answer, but I'm working on it.

Afterword

IT HAS BEEN more than a year since I finished *Gardening for a Lifetime*. Meanwhile, the garden has gone about its quiet business of seasonal change. A warm golden autumn segued into the mild, relatively snowless winter of 2010, during which the vernal pool in the woodland garden remained low. Then, in early March long before the first day of spring, New England was hit by an August heat wave. Primroses were shocked into premature bloom, and daffodils rushed through their all-too-brief season. Even before we turned the clocks ahead to daylight saving time, the grasses and milkweed in the field had begun to shoot up and soon concealed the daffodil foliage.

By June a midsummer night's dream had turned into a nightmare of soaring temperatures and high humidity. For almost three months, the garden lay panting in a stupor of muggy heat. It was the hottest summer on record and one of the driest. Finally, in September, the diminishing winds of hurricane Fiona carried it all away and brought much-needed rain.

Now it is November and next Thursday will be Thanksgiving Day. Contrary to expectations, the fall foliage has been beautiful. At the far end of the garden, fiery leaves still cling to the bare twigs of *Fothergilla gardenii*, and the crescent bed is full of rich autumnal colors. The spiraeas that Erica sheared in July have loosened up into soft globes of golden orange foliage, and the oakleaf hydrangeas have taken on a deep red hue like Moroccan leather.

Events in my life have run parallel to the strange, off-schedule season in the garden. While the inevitable hip surgery went

smoothly on August 31, 2009, and the worn-out joint was replaced with a dashing new titanium model, things began to un-
ravel after Christmas. Out of the blue, a herniated disc in my
back upset my plans for spring.

Instead of being in the garden by March, I was in pain and
walking with the aid of a stick. Weeks of therapy wrought no improvement. Nor were shots of cortisone any more successful. At
least, not at first, but at some point in May, it dawned on me that
I was moving better. So cheered was I by this development that
I ventured into the garden. But the physical therapist had forbid-
den me to bend, lift, or twist, and I soon realized that to garden
without bending, lifting, or twisting was virtually impossible.

Confronted with this new scenario, Erica remained her usual
calm self and went about replacing me. The garden was not a
one-person job. After a couple of unsatisfactory interviews, she
found Kathy Kling, an architect who wanted a change of pace
and loved gardening. The women hit it off at once and from the
first day worked together companionably and with stunning efficiency. All I could do was to make decisions, and even that
seemed difficult.

While I was wrestling with the reality of my physical limitations, an old friend from *Fine Gardening* magazine showed up.
Anita DaFonte is always like a breath of fresh air. She blows in,
usually unannounced and always bearing something delicious
to eat. A truly sublime cook, she spent her teens working side by
side with her father in his bakery and still loves to create things
in the kitchen. On this particular occasion, she unveiled a plum
torte and asked how I was doing. When I told her, she jumped
up from the table where we had been having tea.

"What you need," she said, "is a work party! It would be fun,
like a barn raising. You'd get a whole lot done all at once; everybody would love it. We'd have a great time, and I'd get a chance
to cook!" Anita's warmth and enthusiasm were so contagious

that I soon found myself caught up in the excitement. Erica and Kathy were summoned from the garden.

It was decided that the work party, with Erica as foreman, would assemble at ten o'clock in the morning the following Tuesday, Erica's and Kathy's regular day. Kim Proctor was the first to volunteer her services. Kathy enlisted her sister, Cynthia; I called upon Terence; Anita invited our mutual friend, Jill Chase; and on the day of the work party, Emile Racenet, who had made the beautiful rustic gate to the woodland garden, happened to be in town. He was only supposed to come for lunch, but of course he wound up digging, potting, and planting with the others.

Lunch under the apple tree that day was special, not just because of Anita's superb Spanish tortilla and salad of grilled chicken and fresh baby greens, but because there was something in the air. We were like surfers, lifted out of the ordinary and swept up in a wave of spontaneous goodwill. Poised at the crest, we savored the moment, and the sound of our voices and laughter came back to us, the phenomenon that gave our road its name of Echo Valley.

By three in the afternoon, every last daylily in the crescent bed had been removed and divided. The extra plants were then relocated to other beds or potted up and taken home by anyone who wanted them. In their stead, Emile and Terence planted a dozen small 'Green Velvet' boxwoods.

The improvement was immediate, and the workload had been lightened appreciably. Now there would be no deadheading in July; no ugly bare scapes and tired leaves to clean up in August; no mounds of yellow foliage to cut down in the fall. The tidy forms and shiny evergreen leaves of the boxwoods have already given me five months of beauty and will be a pleasing sight all year. Other than needing water during the drought and a light shearing soon after planting, they have required no care at all.

The work party achieved far more than pushing forward renovations to the garden. It succeeded in shaking me out of my trance of inactivity and changing my attitude. All I had to do was look at the revitalized crescent bed to feel a surge of energy and optimism. Early the next morning I was out in my bathrobe and slippers, taking a hard look at all the flower beds and making a new list of daylily cultivars I could live without. These I marked with a garden stake.

The next week it would be Erica's turn to add plants to the hit list. She and I had become close during the three years she had spent with me. She knew how much I loved the garden and had never made me feel excluded, even when she was doing all the work. Just the same, I was nervous. I had known some of these plants for a long time and was prepared to do battle.

Tuesday rolled around, and we embarked on our walkabout in perfect accord. We had too much *Rudbeckia laciniata* 'Herbstsonne', and the *Artemisia lactiflora* really wasn't worth the space it occupied—the flowers were almost invisible, and the plant had to be staked and retied as it grew to its full six feet. We decided not to fill in any of the spaces where daylilies had been removed but to wait and see what the garden looked like in the spring.

So far so good. But Erica's eyes narrowed when we got to the long border and two vast clumps of peony 'Scarlet O'Hara'. "These," she said, pointing an accusing finger at them, "are a pain in the neck. They bloom for a week and have to be staked three times. What's more, they usually get botrytis." I knew she was right, so with the utmost reluctance I consented to their removal. However, when she began eyeing the river of lamb's ears at the edge of the border, the answer was an absolute, unequivocal "No!" She smiled and shrugged, "It was just a thought."

My own thoughts during the last couple of months have surprised even me. As I can't garden the way I used to, I do a great deal more looking. This kind of looking is as active as hefting a crowbar and much more appropriate. I try to trust my eyes to absorb the essence of the landscape, to take in the big picture, but also to really *see* a single leaf or flower. I discovered this kind of seeing in an essay by Frederick Franck that I read soon after Martin's death.

As a recently qualified oral surgeon, Franck had served on the staff of Albert Schweitzer's jungle hospital in Lambaréné. In an attempt to understand his strange new surroundings, the young doctor began to draw the people and landscape of Africa. In the act of looking and faithfully committing what he saw to paper, he "crawled under Africa's skin." He discovered that when he drew, his attention was so complete that he "'became' that landscape."

Perhaps that will happen to me, too. Off and on, I have drawn and painted since childhood. Drawing could be another way to garden, and there is a lot to see here. Now that most of the perennials, except the ornamental grasses, have been cut down, the leafless trees seem to have backed away from the flower beds, and the sky has opened up.

The lighting effects of November are as dramatic as those of any opera. Shafts of sunlight thrust through roiling navy blue clouds and hit the lawn in flashes of chartreuse. In the low light of early sunset, the faded pink-red walls of the old barn turn to flame and continue to glow even after the sun has disappeared. Then the western sky pales to topaz, and the woodland trees stand out against it as strong black silhouettes.

It will be winter soon. The solstice, when nature shifts gears and the earth stands still, is only a month away. After that, the days will begin getting longer, imperceptibly at first but noticeably by the middle of January. And so it goes on—the cycles, the seasons, the recurring series of changes that make up our lives. That's what it's all about.

Index

About the Author

SYDNEY EDDISON has written six other books on gardening. She has been honored by National Garden Clubs Inc. with their Award of Excellence for 2010. For her work as a writer, gardener, and lecturer, she has also received the Connecticut Horticultural Society's Gustav A. L. Melquist Award in 2002; the New England Wild Flower Society's Kathryn S. Taylor Award in 2005; and in 2006, The Federated Garden Clubs of Connecticut's Bronze Medal. Her garden has been featured in magazines and on television. A former scene designer and drama teacher, Eddison lectures widely and is a frequent contributor to *Fine Gardening* magazine and other publications.